Making Babies

Mary Warnock's work in academic philosophy includes the books *Imagination*, *Memory*, and *Existentialism*, as well as *An Intelligent Person's Guide to Ethics*. Much of her career was spent at Oxford University, and she was later Mistress of Girton College, Cambridge. She was made a Life Peer in 1985, and chaired the Committee of Enquiry into Human Fertilisation and Embryology, whose report formed the basis of legislation in the United Kingdom. Her most recent book is her autobiography, *Mary Warnock: A Memoir*.

Making Babies

IS THERE A RIGHT TO HAVE CHILDREN?

Mary Warnock

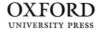
OXFORD
UNIVERSITY PRESS

OXFORD
UNIVERSITY PRESS

Great Clarendon Street, Oxford OX2 6DP

Oxford University Press is a department of the University of Oxford.
It furthers the University's objective of excellence in research, scholarship,
and education by publishing worldwide in

Oxford New York

Auckland Bangkok Buenos Aires Cape Town Chennai
Dar es Salaam Delhi Hong Kong Istanbul Karachi Kolkata
Kuala Lumpur Madrid Melbourne Mexico City Mumbai Nairobi
São Paulo Shanghai Singapore Taipei Tokyo Toronto

with an associated company in Berlin

Oxford is a registered trade mark of Oxford University Press
in the UK and in certain other countries

Published in the United States
by Oxford University Press Inc., New York

British Library Cataloguing in Publication Data

Data available

Library of Congress Cataloging in Publication Data

Data available

ISBN 0–19–280500–2

1 3 5 7 9 10 8 6 4 2

Typeset in New Baskerville
by RefineCatch Limited, Bungay, Suffolk
Printed in Great Britain by
Clays Ltd, St. Ives plc

Contents

Introduction

In this book, I shall address the question of whether people have a right to have children, and in particular whether they can claim a right to receive help in having the children they want. To raise questions about rights is necessarily to enter the domain of morality in a public or social sense. Rights are not simply a matter of individual conscience, for to claim a right is an essentially public act, a demand for justice, or for what is thought to be due to oneself or to others. Yet notoriously, what some may claim as a right, others will argue cannot be a right because they see it as involving what is immoral and therefore as unjustifiable in terms of public policy. There is conflict, for example, between those who argue that a woman has a right to abortion, if this is what she chooses, and those who argue that she cannot claim such a right since abortion involves the destruction of a live human foetus, which is tantamount to murder. And a human foetus, once in existence, has itself a right to life in conflict with the alleged right of the woman to abort it. Similarly, those who claim that someone who is terminally ill has a right to help in bringing her life to an end are countered by those who argue that, however desirable death may be, knowingly to kill or help kill another human being is murder, which is, and must remain, the most serious of all criminal offences. The end, as the Roman Catholics tell us, cannot justify the means. Analogous arguments arise in the increasingly sophisticated field of the birth of children, and it is these arguments that I wish to explore.

Techniques of assisted reproduction

I t goes without saying that people are prone to claim rights most vociferously when they have not got that to which they believe themselves to be entitled. If you have paid for your ticket to get from one place to another and the train stops short of your destination, you may legitimately claim a right to be conveyed somehow or other to where you need to be. Those who claim that they have a right to have children are not likely to be those who already have children, but those who have failed to conceive. My concern, therefore, is in the first place with assisted reproduction. It may be useful to begin by listing the principal methods that can be used to aid conception. The following list and the description of the methods are taken, where appropriate, from the 1985 edition of the Report of the Committee on Human Fertilisation and Embryology, published under the title *A Question of Life* (Blackwell, 1985). This book contains the report, with added comments, of the Government Committee of Inquiry, which had been set up under my chairmanship in 1982 to examine the medical and ethical questions that had arisen after the birth in the UK in 1978 of the first 'test-tube baby', that is a baby born by in vitro fertilization.

First, then, artificial insemination by husband (AIH). This technique is used when a couple have failed to conceive, but the male partner is not completely infertile. It may be thought that the chances of conception would be increased by concentrating the semen, or by inserting it directly into the woman's uterus. (For example, this method may be helpful in overcoming a type of female infertility known as cervical hostility, in which the sperm are damaged or killed by antibodies in the cervical mucus.) There are also situations in which a man may have his semen frozen and stored for later AIH, for example if he is about to undergo treatment such as radiotherapy that may result in sterility. In a case that was notorious at the time, Diane Blood had semen taken from her husband to be frozen while he was in a coma. He did not recover, and she applied to be given AIH after he was dead. She was refused permission by the Human Fertilisation and Embryology Authority (HFEA), the body which, in the UK, has to license all fertility clinics and approve fertility treatments and research. The reason given by the HFEA was that, according to their rules, there had to be written permission from both parents if a child was to be born posthumously. And because Mr Blood had fallen into a coma suddenly (after contracting bacterial meningitis), from which he did not recover, his written permission was not forthcoming. Many people, including myself, thought this an unreasonably strict application of the rules. But the chairman of HFEA, Ruth Deech, believed that posthumous children were bound to suffer psychological trauma, and was adamant in her opposition to Diane Blood's case. I, being a posthumous child myself, took a more lenient view. At any rate, there are no regulations preventing posthumous AIH in Belgium, and so Mrs Blood went there with her husband's preserved semen and conceived a son, who was born in 1998. She now has a second child conceived by the same method. Apart from this particular case, only extremely hard-line moralists see anything ethically objectionable about AIH. For such hard-liners (a small minority), just as it is sinful to engage in sexual intercourse without the intention of procreation, so equally it is a sin to attempt procreation otherwise than by sexual intercourse. The two should be indissolubly linked. Moreover, AIH involves the male in masturbation for the production of semen; and masturbation is held by these extremists to be wrong, whatever its motivation.

Artificial insemination by donor (AID) is used when the male partner is found to be sterile (or it may be used by women who have no male partner, or as part of the procedure of surrogate motherhood, issues to be discussed in due course). There has in the past been strong moral objection to the use of AID. In 1948 the then Archbishop of Canterbury demanded that it be made a criminal offence. In 1960, a UK Committee of Inquiry recommended, more temperately, that it should be strongly discouraged. The use of AID increased, however, and by 1973 a committee was set up in the UK under the chairmanship of Sir John Peel, which recommended that, for the married couples for whom it would be appropriate, AID should be available under the National Health Service, that is, free at the point of delivery for those whose general practitioners had recommended it.

Until the UK Human Fertilisation and Embryology Act of 1990, though a child born by AIH was a legitimate child of the couple, a child born by AID was officially illegitimate. The 1990 Act remedied this disparity, though many thought it wrong to do so—especially those members of the House of Lords who feared that the blood of heirs and successors might thereby be tainted. (For my part, I have to confess a certain sympathy with the objectors. One cannot wholly disregard the genes of a child, though doubtless too much can be made of genetic inheritance.) There have been doubts about the well-being of children born by AID. The difficulties for them stem from the asymmetrical relationship between the parents and the child, who is the biological offspring only of the mother, the father being unknown and, by law in the UK (though not elsewhere in Europe), anonymous. Moreover, there is some doubt about the effect on a family of having a third party involved in the conception of a child, the donor perhaps remaining a shadowy figure in the background of family life.

We come now to more intrusive treatments: first, in vitro fertilization (IVF). This is the procedure by which several eggs are taken from a woman and are mixed in a dish in the laboratory (a 'test-tube') with sperm from a donor (most often her husband) so that fertilization occurs. After a few days, the resulting embryo(s) is inserted into the woman's uterus, where, with luck, it will implant, and she will carry the child to term in a normal pregnancy. When IVF first became a viable treatment for infertility, in the late 1970s, it was thought suitable for only about half of all infertile women, those who had blocked or damaged Fallopian tubes through which sperm could not pass during normal intercourse. Since the 1980s, IVF has been more widely used, not only to remedy infertility but also to enable couples in danger of passing on severe genetic diseases to select only healthy embryos to be implanted in the uterus out of those fertilized in the laboratory.

There were at first three main objections to the use of IVF. The first was the hard-line moral objection that it represented, as did AIH and AID, a deviation from normal sexual intercourse, supposed to be the only justifiable method of procreation. Any other method of procreation was considered morally unjustifiable.

The second objection was based not so much on moral grounds as on grounds of safety. In order to improve the likelihood of success, women about to undergo IVF are commonly given drugs that cause superovulation, the production of more than one egg at each cycle. Several eggs can thus be harvested. All these eggs are then fertilized in vitro, and more than one of the resulting embryos is inserted into the uterus. This increases the risk of multiple pregnancies, rightly regarded as a risk to the health and well-being of the woman and the family. Nevertheless, it seems to be the case that if two or more embryos are transferred to the uterus each helps the other to implant, and this is the justification for implanting more than one embryo at a time.

The third, more deep-seated, and specifically moral objection is that if several embryos are produced in the laboratory and only some of these are transferred to the uterus, the rest will be destroyed, either after having been used for research or immediately. And, as we shall see, there are those who hold that research using human embryos and their subsequent destruction is wrong.

Egg donation is another method of infertility treatment, used when the female partner of a couple is unable to produce her own viable eggs. A mature egg is recovered from a fertile woman donor. This egg is then fertilized in the laboratory, normally using the semen of the partner of the infertile woman. The resulting embryo or embryos are then transferred to the infertile woman's uterus and the pregnancy, with luck, proceeds normally. The resulting child will, this time, be genetically related to the male and not to the female member of the partnership. A significant difference between this procedure and AID is that donating eggs is more risky and involves more intrusion than donating sperm. However, now that eggs may be successfully frozen and used after a period of time (which was not known to be possible in the 1980s) the uses of egg donation are considerably increased. For example, this procedure is sometimes used by women who are about to undergo a medical procedure that may result in sterility or as an 'insurance policy' for those undergoing sterilization or an early menopause; their eggs are taken and preserved for future use.

These, with variants, are the main ways in which assisted conception is attempted. For none of these procedures does there seem to be a generally perceived or agreed moral or prudential objection such as to rule them out of permissible

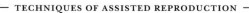

practice. I shall return to the objections that there are, and also discuss the two more generally controversial infertility treatments, surrogacy and cloning, later on.

Who pays?

However, before considering the ethical principles involved in the provision of such assistance, it is necessary to clear away one complicating confusion that results from the particular position of the UK with regard to medical treatment. Ever since the introduction of the National Health Service (NHS), it has been our principle and our pride that treatment should be free to everyone at the point of delivery. And indeed, such free treatment has come to be thought of as itself a right. Failure to deliver adequate free treatment is an increasing source of dissatisfaction in the UK at the present time. This particular source of confusion does not arise, or not in the same form, in countries other than the UK.

To give an example: in Northern Ireland, until the spring of 2001, there were no infertility clinics receiving public funding under the NHS. That year, under the new Parliament at Stormont, the Minister of Health (and incidentally a member of Sinn Fein), opening a meeting of obstetricians and gynaecologists in Belfast, announced that, for at least a two-year experimental period, this policy was to be reversed. Infertility treatment would be available on the NHS. There was great rejoicing among the assembled doctors; and some were heard to say that now at last people in Northern Ireland would get their rights. However, it was not clear to me, by chance present at the occasion, whether they meant the right of access to clinics unavailable hitherto, or the right to free treatment at those clinics. In practice people in Northern Ireland who sought infertility treatment in the form of assisted reproduction before the new edict had mostly come to the British mainland, and had probably had to pay for the treatment they received. Many people would have been unable to do this because they could not afford it.

Increasingly this is a problem over the whole field of medical treatment in the UK: not everything can be afforded. Some people are denied the drugs that would be most effective for their condition on the grounds that the NHS cannot afford them; if they want them, they must 'go private' and pay, not only for the drugs but for their doctor's services as well. We are by now accustomed to the fact that, though there are so-called NHS dentists, in fact only certain categories of patients are entitled to receive free treatment. The rest have to pay. (For example, many NHS dentists will not see a patient who does not agree to go to a hygienist as part of dental treatment; but there is no provision for hygienists' fees to be paid by the NHS.) Similarly, the provision of spectacles, often essential to the well-being of people with bad and perhaps deteriorating sight, is not something that comes free of charge. All this is familiar to people living in the UK, and this type of patient-contribution arrangement is being extended to more and more kinds of medical treatment, many think for the worse. Certainly, the founding fathers of the NHS must turn in their graves.

In the USA, and in most European countries, the position is different. It is expected that people will insure themselves for their medical treatment needs. The issue in this situation is to determine what is and what is not covered by any particular insurance policy. Whatever is not covered must be paid for, or forgone. It is possible, even likely, that private medical insurance, hitherto possessed by a minority in the UK, will become, in some form or another, increasingly necessary. But whatever may in future be demanded in the way of at least partial private insurance policies in the UK, there will remain enormously difficult decisions about what should be the priorities within the NHS, and these problems can only become more acute as medical technology becomes more sophisticated and people's expectations of what it is reasonable to demand as treatment increase. This debate is familiar enough to people living in the UK, and at last is being freely discussed, with greater honesty and openness than before. But the principles involved, though of the greatest importance, are not those I wish to discuss here.

I want instead to consider the question of whether it is the right of everyone to have children, leaving on one side the matter of who pays should medical intervention be necessary to produce those children. Though many people who claim a right to receive medical assistance in reproduction would also claim that they should receive this assistance free in the name of justice, I believe that the two claims can be distinguished, and as far as possible I shall attempt to distinguish them. After all, it would probably be agreed that everyone has a right to dental treatment, even if, in order to exercise that right, they have to pay. This is the same as to say that no one ought to be denied access to a dentist: there is no category of persons deemed to be unfit for dental treatment. Even if a dentist found that he could not treat a particular patient any longer, perhaps because the patient was abusive or violent, the dentist should try as far as possible to ensure that the patient does receive treatment somehow or other. And if a patient was turned away, he might perhaps plausibly claim that his right to treatment had been violated.

The right that no stone should be left unturned

That it is easy to become confused between the claims to a right to treatment on the one hand and a right to free treatment on the other is further illustrated by the case of 'Child B'. This was a case that became notorious in the UK in the middle of the 1990s. There was widespread outrage when the Cambridgeshire Health Authority announced that it would not pay for a third heart transplant attempt for a child, because the cost, weighed against the chances of a successful outcome, did not justify it. The press, predictably delighted by a story that combined the sufferings of a child with the apparent financially motivated callousness of a Health Authority, proclaimed that Child B had been denied the most fundamental right, the right to life. The man who had announced the Health Authority's decision was denounced as a murderer. He later published a calm and brave article, defending himself against the charge and demanding that such decisions be made openly and be seen for what they are: decisions based on priorities, that is value judgements, in which probabilities of outcome must be brought in as a factor, as well as, in this case, the continued suffering of a child who had already suffered very greatly.

The main cause of controversy in the case of Child B was that the decision not to treat her appeared to have been taken on 'purely financial grounds'; it was implied that if her parents had been able to afford private treatment, it would without question have been forthcoming, as of right. The claim of the press was that, given the existence of the NHS, the child had a right to free treatment, on the basis of another right which is taken for granted, namely the right to life. The question of whether it makes sense in all circumstances to claim a 'right to life' was never addressed. Is it reasonable, or even intelligible, to claim a right to something that is impossible? There is, after all, such a thing as futile treatment; and treatment may be judged futile whether it is paid for out of the public or the private purse.

So, to return to the right to have children, if we put on one side the issue of a right to free treatment under the NHS, we may still ask the question whether it makes sense in all circumstances to claim a right to reproduce, where what is at stake is an entitlement to assisted conception. I asked, above, whether it was reasonable, or even intelligible, to claim a right to something impossible. I believe the answer to be 'no'. Have I the right to climb Everest, or to play a violin concerto with the Berlin Philharmonic? I suppose that no one could deny me the right to spend thousands of pounds on trying to do these things, if I were mad enough; but whatever steps I took, I, being me, would not succeed, and in failing I would not have been deprived of a right. Those who are terminally ill have no right to life, however much continued life may be desired for them. Likewise, there will be some couples whose attempts to have children will fail, even with the very best medical help, and, unless there has been gross negligence or incompetence on the part of the medical practitioners involved, these people will not have been deprived of a right, though they may have failed to achieve their hearts' desire. They could not sue their doctor for failing to perform the duty correlative to their alleged right to conceive. He did all he could. In medical contexts, generally, it is important to distinguish between entitlement to treatment, and entitlement to a successful outcome of that treatment. A doctor may properly deem further treatment to be futile, in which case it is time to give up trying. Of course, the more sophisticated and complex available remedies become, the more difficult it may be to come to the old-fashioned conclusion that everything possible has been done. Nevertheless, it seems to me important to remember that, in the context of assisted conception, the only right that could reasonably be claimed would be the right to *attempt* to have a child.

However, bearing this in mind, it is still true that infertility is a condition that can cause extreme misery to those who want to have children, and therefore it is widely, though by no means universally, agreed that the medical profession has an obligation to do what can be done to provide a remedy in the form of assisted reproduction where it is desired, and that research into infertility should be supported. (I shall return later to the question of why it is that some people so desperately want to have children.)

What constitutes a right?

Before examining in more detail the specific claim that there exists a right to assisted conception in an attempt to have children, it is necessary to take a look at the idea of rights in general, in the hope of establishing a clear framework within which to think about the question of principle involved in the particular issue with which we are concerned. A right is an area of freedom for an individual that someone else has a duty to allow him to exercise, as a matter of justice. It is a freedom that one claims, for oneself or for another, and that one can properly prevent other people from inhibiting. So far so good, but we need to consider how the existence of a right is to be established. How is your claim to a right to be upheld? In recent years this has become a highly controversial political issue, especially in the UK since the passage of the Human Rights Act into the Statute Book in 2001. (Before that time, a claim that a British citizen's human right had been breached had to be taken to the International Court at Strasbourg.)

There has been, over the last twenty years or so, a marked change in the concept of rights, at least in the UK; not a sudden change, but a gradual shift in the general understanding of the term. Until about 1960, most people who thought about the matter, or who were interested in legal theory, were broadly speaking adherents of a view known as legal positivism. Following Jeremy Bentham, a philosopher born in the eighteenth century and generally regarded as the founding father of utilitarianism, the legal positivists supposed that a right existed and could be claimed only if there was a law explicitly conferring that right. If a right had been conferred by a law, then some person or persons other than the claimant had a duty to make sure that the right could be exercised, or at least a duty not to stand in the way of its being exercised. It is necessary to insist on this relation between rights and duties, for it is often suggested that if someone has a right then that same person also has a duty. This is not so. If you have a right of way over my land, conferred by a local by-law, it is not you but I who has the duty, a duty to ensure that your way is not obstructed. If the police have a right, conferred by law, to stop and search a suspect, it is the suspect who has the duty to submit to the search, however strongly he may object to it, and to the law that grants such a right to the police.

However, as I shall explain later, there is also a wider sense of the word 'duty' according to which I may have a duty without this implying that you or anyone else has a specific right. And this is where confusion is likely to arise. Thus, a doctor may believe that he has a duty to get up in the night and go to attend a nervous patient, without its being true that the patient has a right to this treatment. The doctor wants to be a good doctor, and his duty, he believes, derives from what a good doctor ought to do. I may feel a strong duty to feed my cat without the cat's having a right to be fed. Such duties are moral duties, and the rights that go with them may perhaps be thought of as moral rights.

It was Bentham's view, frequently expressed, that unless there is a law conferring a right no right can exist. To speak of a right in the absence of a law is 'nonsense on stilts'. This is legal positivism; and it is a view to which, unfashionably, I, on the whole, adhere. Bentham's position was that if you thought that on moral grounds you should be afforded a right which the law does not grant you, then you should argue for the law to be changed, so that it does grant you the right. But until the law is changed you can claim no more than that you ought to have the right, not that you have it. For instance, suppose that a family lives just outside the area within which free transport to school is provided in accordance with a local government ruling; the parent can claim that his child ought to be entitled to free transport just like his neighbour's, that is, that the ruling should be changed. But he cannot claim that, before such a change is made, his child has the right to free transport. All he can do is lobby the authorities and argue for a right to be created that does not at present exist.

One can see from this case why positivism has fallen into disrepute. It seems to give undue authority to the law as it is, and to put on one side considerations of fairness and justice, which the parent of the debarred child would undoubtedly plead. A barrier seems to have been set up between what is broadly speaking fair, and what is legal: between morality on the one hand and the law on the other. A legal system cannot be justified, it is argued, unless it is based on an already existing view of what constitutes a right; and if a law or a ruling is changed, it will be changed according to such a pre-existing criterion of what is due to people. Thus the parent of the debarred child might argue that since his neighbour, who lives only a few hundred yards down the road, is entitled to free transport for her children, it is wrongful and unfair discrimination to debar his child, whose need is identical. He therefore has a right to free transport. The parent could point out, by way of analogy, that the old laws gave masters rights over their slaves. The abolition of slavery recognized the pre-existing right of everyone to be his own master; it did not create such a right.

I believe that to speak of pre-existing rights and of rights under an existing system of law as if they had the same sort of validity leads to confusion. I strongly believe that a system of law must be based on at least some shared moral values; but I would prefer to say, with Bentham, that before the abolition of slavery, slaves ought, on moral grounds, to have had the right to freedom, not that they already had it. For it seems to me that if anyone properly claims a right, it must be appropriate to raise the question where that right came from, what or who conferred it. Rights are part of the structure of a society; in nature, there are neither rights nor duties. If, within a society that accepts the institution of slavery, we hold that slaves none the less in some sense have the right to freedom, we must be appealing to a law other than the laws of that society, a moral law that confers the right to freedom on the slaves. The rights claimed are rights belonging to all human beings in virtue of their humanity, under some universal moral law. And this, of course, is the argument often used. But the content of such a moral law is notoriously vague.

It is sometimes argued, for example, that, apart from the positive laws that currently, and within a particular legislature, create rights, there is a higher law, from which different, higher, universal rights may be derived (and these might include the right of everyone to be his own master, or of everyone to have children). Thus, famously, Sophocles represented Antigone, in the tragedy of that name, determined to do what she conceived as her duty, to show respect for her dead brother by throwing earth on his body, arguing that she had a right to do this though it was forbidden by existing law. In her great speech to Kreon, the Theban tyrant, she invokes a higher law, under which she has not only the right to honour her brother, but the duty to do so.

Antigone's appeal in a way confirms Bentham's view, that without a law there can be no right. If the law that is in force for the time being, in her case under a tyrannical government, has removed what ought to be a right, then her appeal was to a universal and permanent pre-existing law: there must be a law of some kind or other to render the claim to a right intelligible. In our day, implicit or explicit appeals to natural law or natural justice are held to confer natural rights, or universal human rights, one of which, it might be claimed, is the right to have children. There is no positive law in the UK, or, as far as I know, in any other country, that confers on people the right to conceive, or to be helped to conceive.

But it may still be asked what such natural law is, and especially how we come to know what precisely is its content. It is a fundamental principle of justice, one that may indeed be held to be the basis of all positive law, that everyone shall be treated equally, and that no one shall be arbitrarily deprived of what in some sense he needs. But it seems to me plain that this should be referred to as a moral principle, derived from a consideration of the needs and aspirations of human nature. To adopt this way of thinking, that is to regard 'natural law' as a fundamental moral principle (upon which positive laws are doubtless founded and from which they gain their authority), is to distinguish the moral from the legal, while deriving the latter from the former. If someone, for example a slave, or a supporter of abolitionism, claimed a natural or human right to freedom, he would be claiming, for himself or for others, not a legal but a moral right, and invoking a moral principle as the source of this right. He would be asserting that slave-owners had a moral duty to free their slaves. I believe that we should avoid a great deal of confusion if we were to retain the distinction between the legal and the moral, using the language of law and rights for the former, the language of principles and moral obligations for the latter.

However, from the year 2001, with the enactment of the Human Rights Bill in the UK, the option of drawing the distinction between rights as they are conferred by law and general human, or moral, rights has virtually disappeared. I, personally, following the argument above, deplore this move. In 1958 the philosopher Elizabeth Anscombe wrote an article entitled *Modern Moral Philosophy*, in which she put forward the radical argument that the concepts of moral obligation and of moral duty should be abandoned as part of the apparatus of ethics, because such manners of speaking (and thinking) originated from the idea that there were moral laws, or divine commands, that imposed duties and obligations upon people, who were bound to obey these laws. Her contention was that once the belief in divine commands has withered away, as for the most part it has, the language of moral duty and obligation depends for its force on a borrowed sense of authority, which could no longer be rationally justified, nor properly explained, in the absence of its divine source. The expression 'moral duty', uttered in a solemn tone, she argued, appears to carry particular weight, and is used in the hope of motivating action, or inhibiting the satisfaction of certain desires, but, in fact, without its backing of divine command, it is vacuous. It has become nothing but a rhetorical device. She concluded that it would be better, in the business of distinguishing between right and wrong, to go back to an Aristotelian view of human virtue and vice, giving up the fundamentally Christian-based view of obedience to God's commands (though, as she conceded, others than Christians have held such views). This is not the place to go into the details of her argument, with which I do not altogether agree. But I believe that there is a close analogy between what she suggests is the borrowed authority of the expression 'moral duty' and what I hold to be the borrowed authority of the expression 'right' when used outside the framework of specifiable, existent laws. In the absence of a law conferring that right, to claim a right is to employ no more than a rhetorical device.

It is sometimes suggested, and I have indeed hinted already, that the source of human rights is the concept not of law but of need. It might be argued that, at least in a civilized society such as we might aspire to live in, if someone has a need, then this generates a claim on society as a whole that the need should be met (or at least that an attempt should be made to meet it). A government might, for example, be elected on the understanding that no one's needs would be neglected. This was indeed the claim of the 1945 British Labour Government. Does the assertion 'I need x' fare better, then, as a basis for claiming x, than the assertion 'I have a right to x'? Or does it in fact confer a right to x? In one way, this approach may seem promising. For just as to claim a right appears to state a fact, namely that there is a law that confers that right, which can be identified and interpreted, and upheld in court, so to say that some organism needs something seems to be a verifiable statement of fact. And the statement of fact in the latter case seems to be less misleading and equivocal than in the former. It may be a matter of undisputed fact to which all would agree that a particular plant needs a sunny, well-drained site if it is to flourish, or even to survive. However, it is plain that the acknowledgement of this fact does not of itself entail that we ought to provide the plant with such a site. There are some plants we would rather did not flourish, such as dandelions or Japanese knotweed.

Perhaps it is only the needs of human beings that society is obliged to meet, and those individuals correspondingly to have a right that their needs be met. For it may be assumed that we want all human beings (at least within a given society) to flourish (though this in itself is a moral, or at least a political, assumption—a government that questioned it would certainly have difficulty in getting elected). That society had an obligation to meet everyone's needs was, as I have said, the theory behind the welfare state when it was first introduced in the UK in the 1940s. But even at the time, William Beveridge, the founding father of welfarism, recognized that the welfare ideal, that the basic needs of everyone in the country would be met without payment at the point of delivery, would change over time. The concept of what constituted a basic need would change, and claims would escalate. For the idea of a need is generally relative, and this is something that Beveridge understood. Even if one distinguishes between obviously relative needs (such as that I need walking boots if I am to make my attempt on Everest, or a good instrument if I am to try to play my concerto) and 'fundamental' or 'basic' needs, still what counts as a basic need is relative to what is thought to constitute an intolerable way of life if that need were not met. Many people would now regard the possession of a television set as a basic need, on the grounds that life without it would be intolerable. This was obviously not the case in the 1940s.

The judgement of what is or is not an intolerable way of life, the yardstick for the measurement of basic need, is manifestly a judgement about values, though one about which at any one time there is probably a good deal of agreement. Starvation, for example, or severe shortage of water, would be agreed by everyone to be intolerable; and the needs of people who suffer such deprivations may well be seen to be basic, and to generate rights, rights to have their situation remedied. A human being, regarded as a biological organism, will, as a matter of indisputable fact, die without water or food. The threat of death or of torture, of starvation or eviction from one's home, can all be seen as violations of basic human rights, because people cannot flourish without security from such threats. And (though this corollary may make us feel uneasy), it must follow that someone has a duty to see that such basic human rights are not violated, and that everyone's basic needs are met. This duty must fall on someone's shoulders, even though, if we move beyond our own immediate society, it is not clear on whose.

Do people need to have children?

S o we may, after this theoretical preamble, return to the question of whether procreation is a basic need, like nutrition. Well, in one sense plainly it is, for if no one had children, then the human race would not survive, let alone flourish. But, whereas each individual human being needs to eat if he is to survive, not every individual must procreate if he, the individual, is to survive, or even if the human race is to survive. And there are many people who, from deliberate choice or otherwise, do not have children, and who nevertheless flourish as individuals. It seems obvious, therefore, that procreation is not a basic need such as to generate an obligation to satisfy that need in the same way as nutrition.

Could it be argued, however, that, though not everyone wants to have children, for those who do want to, procreation is a basic need, so fundamental as to generate a right? To assert this would be to erode the distinction between relative and basic needs, and indeed to make it impossible to distinguish between heartfelt wishes on the one hand and entitlements on the other, between wants and needs. I am not suggesting that it is always easy to draw this distinction;

we have seen already, in the case of Child B, how the very natural and deep wishes of parents that their child should be given one more chance to live may become translated into the language of rights. There is, of course, some connection between wanting something and needing it. But the relation between them is not straightforward, and falls far short of identity. You may not want some things that you need, and in some cases you may not know what you need, and therefore not want it. And you may want, even want very badly, some things that you do not need. But it is probably impossible not to want any of the things that you need; and there can be no doubt that people who need water, for example, also desperately want it, as long as they retain consciousness. Yet, despite these overlaps, if we allow wanting and needing to slide into each other, with the consequence that there may seem to exist a right to whatever is deeply wanted, then the dangers of the rhetoric of rights, the borrowed authority, escalate.

Some people who claim that everyone (or everyone who wants to) has a right to have children, realizing that it is highly desirable to show where a right comes from, or what confers it, base their claim on Article 16 of the United Nations Declaration of Human Rights promulgated in 1948, and for the most part incorporated in the European Convention of Human Rights. Article 16 starts with the declaration that 'Men and women of full age, without any limitation due to race, nationality or religion, have the right to marry and found a family.' It certainly follows from the endorsement of this article that if, say, Jews or Muslims or couples of mixed race were debarred from having children, or even, perhaps, if no more than one child were permitted to each couple, whatever their race, then a human right would have been infringed. A fundamental principle of fairness would have been contravened. But our concern is not, or not so far, with those who might be *debarred* from having children, on whatever grounds, but with those who are *unable* to have children without assistance, and our question is whether they have a right to that assistance.

Can there be a right to do what is morally wrong?

There are some people who argue, as we have seen, that there cannot be a right to treatment for infertility involving assisted conception, since such treatment is itself morally wrong; and there can be no moral right to something that is, or involves, moral wrong-doing. As I have already said, such an assertion is often abbreviated into the slogan 'The end cannot justify the means'. The most extreme form of such arguments, put forward by some but by no means all Roman Catholics, is, as I have mentioned, that infertility treatments such as AIH, AID, or IVF depend on male masturbation for the production of sperm, and that masturbation is a sin, whatever its intended outcome. Therefore such treatments are intrinsically sinful. A variant of this extreme argument is that since the sole justification of sexual intercourse is reproduction, it must follow that reproduction cannot be permitted without sexual intercourse (this is a dubious logical step; it might moreover be argued that, if sexual intercourse is itself barely to be morally tolerated, it would be better to do without it, and reproduce always by the indirect process of IVF, or even asexually, by cloning).

A less extreme argument that IVF is wrong relates to the fact that it requires further research in order to improve its success rate. When IVF first became available as a potential remedy for some forms of infertility, its success rate was so low that it was essentially an experimental procedure; it would certainly have been fraudulent to offer it as a treatment with a good chance of a successful outcome. Research into the procedure of IVF demands that live human embryos should be produced in the laboratory by the introduction of egg to semen in the 'test-tube' and their development be monitored, among other things to find the best way to mirror the environment of the human uterus and increase the likelihood of successful fertilization and development. The embryos used in such experiments would not be subsequently inserted into a woman's uterus, but would be destroyed. This process, according to the powerful 'pro-life' lobby (mainly, but not exclusively, Roman Catholic), is morally wrong. This argument is akin to arguments against abortion: in both cases the embryo (or foetus) is endowed with an inviolable 'right to life'. Someone who demands IVF treatment as a right is, on this view, overlooking the conflicting right to life of all embryos brought into existence during the procedure. Not all of them will be inserted into a uterus; some will inevitably be destroyed.

The moral status of the human embryo

We come here to the crux of the case against research using human embryos, a necessary condition, as I have argued, of the provision of most infertility treatments. The question centres on the status that should be accorded to the human embryo at the earliest stage of its development. The so-called pro-life group argue that at the moment of conception (however this 'moment' is to be identified) a human being, complete with human soul and potential human body, comes into being. One should therefore no more destroy an embryo at this stage of its development than one should destroy a later foetus or indeed a child or adult. All such acts of destruction are forms of murder.

Some scientists working in the field of infertility research were genuinely amazed by this argument. For example, the eminent physiologist Dame Anne McLaren, head of the UK Medical Research Council Mammalian Unit in the 1980s, later wrote to me that 'up till that time [the time of the Government Committee on Human Fertilisation and Embryology, of which she was a member] I had led an ethically sheltered existence, and it had never crossed my mind that fertilising frozen and thawed donated human eggs as part of a research project to help young women [to conceive] could equally well be described as "creating in order to destroy"'. For the pro-life group held that there was something especially horrendous in deliberately 'creating' a human being only then to deprive it of its chance of life, by failing to place it in a human womb, but instead throwing it down the sink.

Underpinning the pro-life objection to research using early embryos is the belief that there is a specific moment when human life begins. Sperm and eggs, though human and alive, do not count as 'human life' in the sense required; it is only when they have come together that a human individual is created who has the potential to become a human person. This belief, though now often couched in terms of the individual's DNA, already incorporated in the cells making up the embryo, in fact owes a good deal to Aristotle, who not only had no notion of DNA, but did not even know of the existence of human eggs, speculating that an embryo was formed by male sperm somehow thickening female blood within the uterus. He held that a human being begins to exist when the specifically human form of life enters the embryo, at a fixed date, earlier for males than females. There were three kinds of life or soul; the vegetative, shared by all living things, including plants; the sensitive, shared by all animals, including man; and the rational, peculiar to man. When Aristotle's speculations were discovered and taken over, first by Thomas Aquinas and later as the official doctrine of the Church, there was much discussion of the exact timing of this entry of the human life, or soul, into the body. Of course by now the concept of 'the soul' had entirely changed since the

days of Aristotle, the soul being now a thoroughly Christian-
ized entity, immortal, and in a special sense in the hands of
God, and of infinite value. It was gradually agreed that one
could not be sure of the exact time at which ensoulment took
place, and therefore, to be safe, it must be assumed that it was
at the moment of conception, or fertilization. It followed that
from this moment on, the growing embryo must be
regarded, like other human beings, as possessed of a 'sacred'
life, to be protected at all costs from destruction. This cluster
of beliefs accounted for the question most frequently asked
by those who wanted to decide whether research using
human embryos was justified, namely the question 'When
does life begin?' Some people argued that there should be a
moratorium on all such research until scientists could answer
this crucial question. But it was a question misleadingly for-
mulated. It sounded like a scientific question, but was in fact
a moral question in disguise: 'At what stage does an embryo
become morally significant?'

Non-Aristotelian, Darwinian biologists could not accept
the view that human beings spring into existence at a particular moment. The then Archbishop of York, John Habgood,
put the point very clearly in the debate on the second
reading of the Human Fertilisation and Embryology Bill
(Hansard, 7 December 1989). He said 'Scientists in general
and biologists in particular deal mostly in continuities and
gradual changes from one state to another. This is true of
evolution, in which the transition from the pre-human to
the human took place over countless generations. There was
never a precise moment when it could have been said, "Here

is a hominid and here is a man". But this is not to deny that as a result of the process there emerged a profound and indeed crucial set of difference between hominids and men. The same is true of individual lives. . . . It seems strange to a biologist that all the weight of moral argument should be placed on one definable moment at the beginning.' And he went on to say (doubtless to the alarm of fundamentalists) 'Christians are no more required to believe that humanness is created in an instant than we are required to believe in the historical existence of Adam and Eve.'

The Bill drew a distinction between the embryo before and after fourteen days from the time when fertilization was established in the laboratory. Before fourteen days, the embryo, or pre-embryo as it was scientifically known, was a loose cluster of first two, then four, then sixteen cells, undifferentiated. An undifferentiated cell could develop into any of the types of cell that go to make up the human body, and some of them would not become part of the embryo at all, but would form the placenta or the umbilical cord. After fourteen days, there begin to appear the first traces of what will become the central nervous system of the embryo, the primitive streak (or the two primitive streaks, since at about this time identical twins may be formed). From this time the cells develop into their particular types, and the embryo develops fast into a recognizable foetus (or foetuses). There are therefore good scientific reasons for distinguishing between an embryo before fourteen days, when it can hardly be referred to as a human individual, and an embryo after this stage. A different status was accorded on the basis of these developmental differences. A human embryo was allowed to be kept alive in the laboratory, and used for research, up to fourteen days from its established fertilization. To keep an embryo alive longer became a criminal offence, subject to up to ten years imprisonment. The more developed the embryo, the more its proper treatment was deemed to approach to the treatment of a human individual.

Such arguments as these prevailed, and the Bill became law in the UK in 1990. Though there are still those who think that research using pre-fourteen day live human embryos and their subsequent destruction is morally wrong, generally people have now come to take it for granted, and moreover to regard it as something that has enormous potential for the good of those who are infertile, as well as for increasing knowledge of the early development of the human embryo, knowledge that can be put to numerous beneficent uses. IVF has become almost a routine procedure, though its success rate is still not satisfactory. In the year 2001 the permitted scope of research using pre-fourteen day embryos was widened by Parliament to include areas other than infertility. Stem-cell research was now permissible under the law. Such research involves using embryos in the laboratory as a source of undifferentiated cells, which can be induced to develop into any one of the types of cell that make up the human body, with the ultimate aim of using therapeutic cell transplant to treat a variety of conditions from Parkinson's disease to certain types of childhood leukaemia. So the argument that no one can have a right to treatment depending on such research because of its intrinsic wrongness must, I think, be dismissed. Parliament, at least, has twice decided that embryo research is permissible.

This ruling, of course, applies only in the UK. Elsewhere in Europe, research using live embryos as part of infertility treatment, though illegal in Germany, is generally permitted elsewhere. However, it is only in the UK, so far, that embryonic stem cell research is permitted. In the USA there is no federal funding either for IVF and related treatments or for the development of new cell-lines for medical research. By some extraordinary muddle, President George W. Bush, at the beginning of his administration, decided to allow research using the few stem-cell lines that had already been isolated. But these, it turns out, are neither all accessible nor all particularly useful for medical advances. The absence of federal funding does not, however, prevent privately funded clinics or commercial companies from carrying out research. While by the legislation of 1990 in the UK all research, however funded, must be licensed by the Human Fertilisation and Embryology Authority, a statutory body set up by the 1990 Act, in the USA there is no regulation applying across the board.

Back to infertility

However, despite all the advances in embryology and genetics we still seem no nearer to an answer to the question of whether or not people have an actual right, capable of being proved, to the provision of assisted conception. Let us therefore descend from the regions of high abstraction, from talk of rights and correlative duties, of what does or does not constitute a basic human need, or a consequent human right, of when a human becomes an individual to be considered of moral significance, and consider the matter from ground level. It is certainly the case, as I have already said, that infertility is a malfunction that can cause acute misery. Though some infertile couples seem able to get over their disappointment in failing to conceive, there are others whose lives are blighted. Their entire picture of their future has been disrupted; they may feel that they are deprived of what gives meaning to the lives of their contemporaries and was to have given meaning to theirs. Their whole life-plan was founded on the idea of a family, and they have been frustrated.

It is difficult to analyse this acute longing to have children on the part of some of those who fail to conceive, though it is, for me at least, extremely easy to sympathize with it. It is not enough, as I have suggested, to put it down to a purely biological urge, since increasingly large numbers of people, even if they live together as a couple, make a deliberate decision not to start a family. These couples are self-sufficient; their careers, their interests, their travels are enough to give meaning to their lives. Nor are they necessarily those who simply do not like children, and are not prepared, therefore, to put themselves out to have them. It should have been obvious, ever since contraception became readily available, that couples could choose not to have children, and that those who do make this decision are not to be treated as 'unnatural', or somehow less than fully human. Their chosen way of life is perfectly morally acceptable. But, morally acceptable or not, there are those who find it impossible to accept it as their own.

In the British newspaper the *Observer* in June 2001, Laurie Taylor and his son Matthew published an article contrasting the numbers of people who do not want children now with the numbers in the 1960s, when Matthew Taylor was born. The contrast is even more stark if one contrasts the numbers with those ten years earlier, after the Second World War, when those of us who started our marriages and our careers simply assumed that we would have children, and that this was to be the fulfilment of our joint lives. Then, it was almost universally true that failure to conceive caused deep disappointment and distress. But even if it has become more generally socially acceptable to remain childless, it still remains true that the desire to have children may for some become an obsession. And the psychological distress is particularly hard to bear because, except in a minority of cases, a couple cannot know for certain that they are not going to conceive. They may continue to hope, as the months go by, and be endlessly disappointed. It is becoming increasingly difficult to find babies to adopt, as the stigma attached to single motherhood diminishes. In any case, adopting a baby is for many people an intolerable risk. As we become more aware of the role of inherited genes in the character of our children, so the bringing up of children in no way genetically connected to us has come to seem a quite different undertaking from that of bringing up a child who shares our own genes. It may be worthwhile, but it is not the same. At any rate, when the Committee of Inquiry into Human Fertilisation and Embryology was deliberating in the mid-1980s they had no difficulty in agreeing that for those who wanted children, infertility merited treatment, and that scientists and the medical profession would be right to continue to develop remedies through research and practice; and that those who need assistance in conceiving ought to be provided with access to such assistance.

The Committee had been set up after the birth of the first 'test-tube baby' by IVF. The techniques were new, and the success rate of IVF was very low. One of the questions before the Committee was whether research in the field should continue, and if so how it should be regulated. On the matter of regulation, it was quite difficult to reach agreement; but on the fundamental issue of whether research, without which treatment could not honestly be offered, was warranted, we, the committee members had no doubts. No arguments, though they were sometimes put to us, about overpopulation in the world as a whole had any bearing on whether individual people who were suffering from a condition that might be capable of remedy (and who would after all form a tiny proportion of all the people in the world) should be helped if possible to become parents. There is always a great difficulty in bringing general or global arguments to bear on individual cases. It was obvious that for a couple in genuine distress over their childlessness, it would be of no comfort whatever to tell them that the world is overpopulated, and so they should be glad. They do not care about the population of India, they want to remedy the emptiness of their own nursery.

Some people, I suppose, want children in order to relive some of their own childhood experiences. I am sure that this was part of my pleasure in my children, if not of my motivation for having them. Others, on the contrary, want to be able to do better by their children than their own parents did for them.

But the most obvious basis for the longing to have children is, perhaps, a kind of insatiable curiosity: what will the random mixture of genes produce? What will be familiar, what unfamiliar? The amazing pleasure of each child is that he or she is new, a totally unique being that has never existed in the world before, seeing things with his own eyes, saying things that are his own inventions. It is, for me, easy to appreciate why seeing other people experience these delights that you so much long for may become intolerable.

So, in the most general terms, the Committee agreed with the humane principle of the medical profession, that it would be wrong, on compassionate grounds, not to offer assisted conception to those who sought to overcome their infertility, in other words that the medical profession had a duty, in the wider sense already noted, to continue to provide assistance. For doctors generally agree that it is their duty to try to alleviate suffering and to discover and if possible treat its cause, and so it is with infertility. The question of rights hardly arises. For, as a general rule, doctors may believe it to be their duty (in the broad sense) to treat a particular condition, without their patients having to claim a right to treatment, only a wish to be treated and a willingness to cooperate.

May doctors refuse treatment?

Yet it was clear to the Committee that some doctors wanted the freedom to turn away some applicants for infertility treatment, despite their general duty to provide treatment. And so the matter of rights arose in a somewhat different form. On what grounds might a couple aspiring to assisted conception be refused it? Once again, in asking this question, I will try to distinguish between issues that might arise within the context of the National Health Service, and those that might arise in private clinics, in the UK or elsewhere, in other words those that turn on principles not linked to scarcity of resources or distribution of health care.

It was obvious to us that a consultant might use his clinical judgement to turn away an aspiring couple if he concluded that no form of assisted conception he could provide would work for them (in other words, that treatment would be futile) or that for some reason their own health would be badly affected by such treatment. In such cases, he would probably, and in my view rightly, offer them the chance of a second clinical opinion. But there was an eminent and by then elderly member of the Committee, herself an obstetrician, who said that she would turn away other couples whom she thought to be 'unsuitable'. When asked how she would explain to them her decision that they were unsuitable, she replied that she would simply tell them that in rejecting their application for treatment, she was exercising her clinical judgement, as she was entitled to do. As chairman of the Committee, I found this a morally objectionable line to take, unless, as there well might be, there were genuine clinical doubts about whether the pregnancy, if it were achieved, would be deleterious to the health of the woman, and I pressed her hard for some account of what would be her criteria for 'unsuitability', but without success. She could not, or did not care to, distinguish between clinical and what I suspected were social or moral tests of unsuitability.

In the course of a later meeting, another practising gynaecologist, an extraordinarily humane man, devoted to his patients and they to him, sought the advice of the Committee on whether he should offer IVF treatment to a couple who were infertile, and both of whom were blind. This led to a prolonged discussion, and of course took us back to the possibility of finding general non-clinical criteria of 'suitability for treatment'. The case of the blind couple presented few difficulties. They were intelligent people, they had rationally considered the problems they would face in bringing up a child, and what help they could obtain to ease those problems, and they deeply wanted children. The problems they would have were their problems, not those of their consultant. At this point, the inevitable objection was raised: it's all very well for the consultant to help his patients to get what they want and achieve a successful birth, but what about the good of the child? After all, in any case involving infertility, there is besides the patients a potential third party to be considered, the hoped-for child, whose interests, it is generally held, must not be overlooked, indeed must come first. So the principle has been enunciated, and is indeed included in the 1990 Fertility and Embryology Act, as well as in the guiding principles of the Human Fertility and Embryology Authority set up under that Act, that *the good of the child is paramount.* Yet what exactly this principle means, what force it has, and how the child's future good is to be estimated have not been seriously examined, nor did we on the Committee examine such issues. The principle sounded good, and we adopted it.

Instead of going in for further analysis of what, if anything, would determine whether certain patients might be deemed 'unsuitable for treatment' on other than clinical grounds, we invented a situation in which a couple seeking assisted conception had, one or both of them, a proven history of child abuse. (We did not go into the question of how the consultant came to know this: we were dealing, after all, with a hypothetical case, an extreme example, by which to test the concept of 'non-clinical unsuitability' and 'the good of the child'.) The eminent woman obstetrician still maintained that she would examine the couple and tell them that they were too old, or whatever other pseudo-clinical reason she could think up for refusing them treatment. The rest of us held, more tentatively, that the couple should not be given treatment, but should be told the true reason, and offered the opportunity to see whether another consultant might take a more lenient view. We took the question with us on a visit we had arranged to meet some doctors in Belfast, and I put the question to them. One of them spoke up with a great air of certainty and said 'I should counsel them'. So I persisted, and asked what he would do if they claimed a right to treatment; he said, slightly more hesitantly, 'I would counsel them and counsel them until they went away'. He was a fierce little man, and I felt sure that if it had been me I would have gone away fairly quickly. Nevertheless, he did not seem to me to have produced a wholly satisfactory answer.

One reason for my doubt on this point is that, perhaps, people can and do change. In other spheres, previous offences are not allowed to stand against people's names forever. Furthermore, one cannot always wholly rely on verdicts of child abuse. Finally, though I would think that a consultant who had turned away this hypothetical couple had probably chosen rightly, and was perhaps entitled to exercise what would be a social or moral rather than a clinical judgement of the case, I would be uneasy about any suggestion that one could derive from this example a set of criteria by which to judge social or moral 'suitability' for infertility treatment. Even if, as he almost certainly would, the consultant discussed the issues not only with medical colleagues, but with psychiatrists, social workers, prison officers, and others, it would still seem to me very rash if he, or the clinic in which he worked, were to try to generalize from the particular case, and lay down rules under which patients might be excluded. Rather, all new dubious applicants should be examined on the merits of their own case.

Applicants might, after all, have very different motives for desiring assisted conception. For example, a woman might seek treatment after she has had several children and has been sterilized at her own request. Let us suppose that she has married for a second time, and now very much wants to bear the child of her second husband. Some would argue that since she has children, albeit from a former marriage, she is not entitled to treatment designed for the infertile. Bearing in mind, however, that we are not concerned with free treatment, and are therefore not dealing with issues of fair distribution of scarce resources, it would seem harsh to refuse her treatment on the grounds that she had deliberately brought herself to the position of being infertile. There seems nothing in principle wrong with treating her, and certainly no argument derived from the idea of the good of the child would suffice. She might be an admirable parent.

But there are undoubtedly more controversial cases. There has recently been a good deal of press coverage of cases in which postmenopausal women—infertile, certainly, but on account of their age—have been given assisted conception. There is an Italian doctor, Professor Severino Antinori, an IVF pioneer, and now an advocate of human cloning, who has at least once assisted such a birth. He was approached in the year 2000 by a sixty-two-year-old French woman, hitherto childless, who wanted to have a child, with the help of donated semen and egg, by means of IVF. Though she did not tell him this, the sperm donor in this case was to be her brother. He turned her down for treatment, largely on the grounds of suspicion about her psychological condition. She, with her brother, thereupon went to Los Angeles, where, still concealing the fact that the donor was her brother, she asked for and obtained IVF treatment and gave birth successfully to a healthy son. (At the same time, as a kind of fail-safe, a surrogate mother, the egg donor, had been impregnated with the brother's semen and also gave birth to a baby, a girl, who is being brought up with the boy, by the sixty-two-year-old woman and her brother.) This bizarre case caused outrage in France, where it was labelled 'social incest'. In any case, in France it is illegal to give assistance for a postmenopausal woman to conceive, the law being based on the concept of the good of the child, as well as on a widely shared feeling expressed in the statement that 'there is a time to be a mother and a time to be a grandmother', and that such late births contravene that common-sense law. In this particular case in France, in which there was a history of appalling family discord over the inheritance of property, it seems that the motive for having these two babies was so that the estate should not pass out of the immediate family (who had hitherto, apparently, been on the worst of terms). I have no doubt that in the UK, and probably in most other countries, the woman's application for IVF treatment would have been turned down, if only because the motivation for having the babies seems to have been purely financial; the babies were being created for the sake of settling potential family disputes. Anthony Trollope would have understood the deep importance in some families of having an heir to property: the chanciness of bringing this off, and the resignation that must be adopted when Nature has not produced an heir, is there in the background of many of his novels. The supposition that whatever age a woman is she can demand treatment to allow her to bear an heir to her property is totally alien to this somewhat romantic view of the chances of birth and death. Yet, though not wholly rational, such views are deeply held and deeply felt, and cannot be easily swept aside simply because a new technology makes it possible for an older woman to conceive.

Most infertility clinics in the UK have an upper age limit for treatment well below sixty-two, and this is a matter of policy, broadly based on considerations of the health of the mother and the good of the child (especially when he is growing up, when his aged mother may become a tremendous burden, a responsibility, and a source of guilt and embarrassment), which amount to non-clinical, or at least not entirely clinical, reasons for rejecting an applicant. I believe that even without laying down strict criteria for accepting or rejecting patients, it should be possible for a doctor or a clinic to say 'no' in such cases, and, as I have suggested, to give the real reason: 'it does not seem right'. A doctor might feel that he could not conscientiously treat such a patient. The most he could do would be to advise her to go abroad for treatment, to Italy perhaps, or to the West Coast of America where private clinics flourish and where there is no state or federal regulation of what can be tried, as long as it is paid for.

I believe that, though it would be impossible to lay down in advance all the cases that might arise, and all the criteria that should be used to rule them out or in, infertility treatment is an area in which problems will not arise all that often; we should be content to work within the general framework of provision of assisted conception services to those who need them. In the vast majority of cases, the refusal of treatment will be based on genuinely and straightforwardly clinical judgement. In a few cases, non-clinical judgements may be involved (and doctors will never like making them). I shall return to the matter of such non-clinical judgement in due course.

The slippery slope

In the meantime, I would say only that, while I am on the whole not much enamoured of the 'slippery slope' argument, I am inclined to fall back on a version of it here. Generally, the slippery slope argument, which has an equal appeal to the conservative and to the sensational press, takes the following form: x is a step towards y, z, etc.; x is not perhaps especially undesirable in itself, but y and z certainly are; and once x has been permitted, y and z will inevitably follow. Thus it may be argued that while it may not be absolutely wrong to abort a foetus discovered to be grossly damaged, if this is permitted then it will be impossible to prevent abortion on more trivial grounds, such as that the foetus is of the non-preferred sex, that it will have a mild disability if it is born, that it will have some other undesired characteristic. By allowing abortion of a severely damaged foetus, we would be on the highroad to eugenics. And if we allow ourselves to start on that road, we will end up sending whole groups of people whom we regard as undesirable to their deaths in the gas chamber. Therefore, we must prohibit abortion of a grossly damaged foetus. The rallying cry of those who deploy the slippery slope argument is 'Where will it end?'

The trouble with the argument lies in the word 'inevitably'. There is no logical connection leading from x to y or z. In the case of using early embryos for experimental purposes— where the slippery slope exponents had a field day, envisaging Frankenstein's monsters brought to birth in the laboratory—allowing that scientists may keep an embryo alive in the laboratory for fourteen days does not logically entail that they will keep it alive for longer. In this case, a block was placed on the slope by legislation. To keep an embryo alive in the laboratory longer than fourteen days from fertilization was made a criminal offence; and no one working in the field of embryology would wish to incur a prison sentence. His entire career would be brought to an end.

The supposed inevitability of y and z following from x seems more a matter of human propensities than of logic. If you give a concession to someone, they will want more. Give them an inch and they will take an ell. And this, or something like it, is what I fear if consultants are given the right to turn away applicants for assisted conception on other than clinical grounds, grounds of social or moral 'suitability for treatment'. I do not suppose that most consultants want to make such non-clinical value judgements; but some might want to, and might fall into the way of judging applicants for treatment to be too feckless, say, or too stupid or too frivolous, or too otherwise undesirable, even of the wrong race or colour, to merit treatment. There is, after all, thankfully no test that people have to pass to entitle them to have children by the normal means. (Though it must be admitted that the intellectually disabled, or others who seem unable to avoid pregnancies, are sometimes recommended for sterilization, with or without consent. But this generally produces an out-cry, rightly, in my view.) One might ask, therefore, why assisted conception should be any different. The children of assisted conception may not always flourish, and may need in some cases to be taken from their parents and fall to the care of the State. But we have no idea how many such children there are; and in any case the same is true of the children of normal conception. It seems to me misleading to argue, as some have, that if children are deliberately brought into the world through the 'artificial' means of IVF or AID there is an extra duty to ensure that they will flourish. Even if there were such a duty it could not fall on the consultant; he is not per-sonally responsible for the future well-being of the children he helps to deliver. The duty must lie, as it always does, with the parents of those children; and if they fail in their duty, then, as is regularly the case, society must take over.

Interim conclusion

I conclude, therefore, that while conception cannot be regarded as a fundamental right, nor as a universal need generating a right, and while there is certainly no positive law conferring on everyone the right to have children, nevertheless the infertile who want to conceive are entitled to expect that they will be given the medical assistance they need, even if they have to pay for it. Further, I conclude that while in some extreme cases consultants or clinics may refuse to treat infertile individuals on grounds other than clinical unfitness, these cases are likely to remain rare, each should be judged on its own merits, and the grounds for turning the would-be patient away should be openly declared.

Are those who are not infertile entitled to assisted conception?

Not all those who seek assisted conception are infertile. For example, now that women are becoming increasingly ambitious, and successful in careers that are not easily combined with pregnancy and motherhood, they may seek either to have their husbands' sperm frozen for later use in AIH or to have embryos created in the laboratory, using their eggs and their husbands' semen, while they are still young and at the height of their fertility. These embryos could then be frozen, and kept until the mother was ready to become pregnant and start a family. On the Committee of Inquiry to which I have already referred, alongside the infertile child-abusing couple, we invented the case of the fertile successful ballerina, who wanted to postpone raising her family until her days of stardom were over. Should she have access to treatment, not to overcome infertility but to help her to combine motherhood with a necessarily shortish, intensely active career, safeguarding herself and her husband against the increased risks associated with conceiving a child in middle age, or against the risk of late-onset infertility? Unless one belongs to the minority who regard IVF as itself morally wrong, there seems no reason to hold that the ballerina should not seek treatment, if she is prepared to pay for it, and risk an unsuccessful outcome. (For IVF is still less likely to lead to a pregnancy than normal intercourse and the older the patient undergoing IVF, the less are the chances of success. AIH is equally less likely to succeed if the would-be mother is in her 40s.)

Another circumstance in which a couple who are not infertile may seek IVF treatment is when any child they have together is at high risk of suffering from a serious heritable disease. In such cases, several embryos may be created in the laboratory, and only those not affected by the disease implanted in the woman's uterus (or, for example, if the disease is haemophilia, which affects only males, only female embryos will be implanted). There has also been a controversial case in the UK in which the parents of a child in urgent need of a bone marrow transplant sought to have another child by IVF to act as a donor, there being no other available source of compatible bone marrow for the operation. In the proposed procedure, several embryos would be created in the laboratory using the eggs and sperm of the sick child's parents, and the embryo whose genetic material was compatible with its sibling would be chosen for implantation so that it could later become a donor, thereby saving the life of its sibling. This case provoked a storm of controversy, on the grounds that the newborn baby would be used as a means to an end, and therefore would be valued only as a means, rather than as an individual in its own right. I cannot, myself, see any objection to this procedure. The baby who would be born would be loved, but not only as the saviour of its sibling.

It might indeed be doubly precious, both simply for existing as babies should be, and as having been the saviour of another life. After all, existing children in a family sometimes give, say, a kidney to save a sibling, and they are loved and honoured for doing so. The objection to the procedure in this case was that it would lead to 'designer babies', children born to fulfil some wish of their parents and not therefore valued intrinsically or for their own sake. Though, reluctantly, I have made use of the slippery slope argument myself, I do not in this case see that there exists such a treacherous slope. There is no precedent here for a frivolous use of IVF for the selection of desirable embryos for implantation. The saving of a life is not a frivolous matter. Nor is there any reason to suppose that, if the life of the existing child could not be saved, the newborn baby, who it was hoped would provide the means to save it, would be rejected, or any the less loved. Probably the reverse would be true. As usual, every case needs to be looked at on its own merits and in its particular context. In the end the judgement against this family was overthrown at appeal.

However, perhaps the most contentious cases in which treatment is sought for reasons other than infertility are those of homosexuals of both genders who request assisted conception, individually or as a couple. Of course, a consultant or a clinic may declare as a policy that only heterosexual couples will be treated, whether they are fertile or infertile. This would be to deny that there was any duty to treat everyone who applied, and thus to deny that everyone has a right to be helped to have a child. The consultant would be saying, in effect, 'you may think you have a right to have a child. I disagree'; and he might tell the would-be patient to try to find another practitioner who would share his or her view that a right exists. As I have said, there is no positive law that confers on people the right to have children; but neither is there a law that forbids homosexuals to have children.

Is one *entitled* to do anything not prohibited by law? Well, of course it depends what one means by 'entitled'. There are some things which would be generally agreed to be morally wrong, but which are not criminal offences—many kinds of deception, for example, or ill-treatment at a domestic level. In such cases it seems to me, as I have already argued, that to talk about rights introduces confusion. The question must be whether such things are indeed morally wrong, and, if they are, on what grounds they are held to be so. Suppose a wife constantly injures her husband by speaking ill of him behind his back, or by making him seem foolish, or by deceiving him about what money from their joint account is spent on. All of these ways of behaving could well be regarded as morally offensive. Even if the husband were provoked into saying that in marriage he had a right to expect better from his wife, this would be only a moral entitlement, though he might use it as a moral justification for seeking divorce. The basis of the moral judgement would be that marriage is supposed to be mutually supportive, that a spouse is not supposed to act as an enemy. These are the moral values built into the institution of marriage; they give rise to reasonable expectations, admittedly often disappointed, but not to criminal proceedings. A horrible wife may be generally morally condemned, but not prosecuted simply on the grounds that she is horrible.

Because of the lack of precision in moral claims such as those of the husband in our example, some people have advocated drawing up a more specific contract before marriage, which might give rise to accusations of breach of the contract in some particular circumstances or the violation of specific rights. I cannot believe that such contracts would be very helpful, even if they did lend some colour to the claim 'I had a right to expect . . . '. The difficulty is that morality, unlike the law, is, in David Hume's words 'more felt than thought on', as much a matter of sentiment as of reason. This means that the nice and the nasty are as morally significant as the right and the wrong. The horrible wife described above is simply a nasty person; and no one can claim it as a *right* that someone else should be nice, much as they might wish them to be.

Once again, then, I want to emphasize the distinctness of the moral and the legal, and this was the point of the above example. People may inflict on one another moral injuries, sometimes very serious injuries, without breaking any law that prohibits them from behaving as they do. The relevant question is this: if it is conceded that homosexuals have no positive legal right to have children (as no one has), but equally they are not legally prohibited from having them, is it morally permissible to offer them assistance in reproducing, even though they are not infertile?

There is one factual matter to be noted here, as a preliminary to considering the question: artificial insemination can be carried out at home, with a syringe, and without medical intervention. Lesbians who want to become pregnant

can persuade a man, perhaps himself homosexual, to provide semen, and when they become pregnant can present
themselves to an antenatal clinic as an unmarried mother,
the father of the child having gone away. The pregnancy and
birth will then be managed in the ordinary way (in the UK,
probably by the NHS). Similarly, though doubtless with
rather more difficulty, male homosexuals could find someone willing to carry their child, who would act as a surrogate,
having inseminated herself with their donated semen, and,
once again, when she became pregnant she would present
herself to an antenatal clinic as an unmarried mother, the
father of the child having disappeared. The fact that homosexuals can start their families without medical intervention,
as long as they can persuade someone to provide semen or to
provide a womb, means that those who really want to have
children will do so anyway, whether other people think it
morally wrong or not. There are, however, enormous advan-
tages in having AID properly carried out, and, especially for a
lesbian couple who want a child, the safeguard of screening
of semen at a clinic set up for this purpose is obviously desirable. It is better to have properly regulated than unregulated
assisted conception. And so the question is whether this particular kind of assisted conception should be available to
everybody, regardless of his/her sexual orientation and
regardless of whether any resulting child will be brought up
by a homosexual couple. I do not believe that there is any
reason to prohibit such a family arrangement. (Nor do I
believe that the number of homosexuals applying for assisted
conception will ever be very great.)

Such an outcome will seem outrageous to many people. They will argue that consideration of the good of the future child should absolutely prohibit homosexual couples from having and bringing up children. As a further development in the passionate debate in the UK's House of Lords about the notorious Clause 28 of the Learning and Skills Bill, in the summer of 2000 Baroness Young and many of her supporters argued that for teachers to present homosexuality as an option, a possible and accepted alternative way of life, was to undermine the family, corrupt young people, and lead them into disastrous and permanently damaging experiments. How much worse such moralists must think it if not merely teachers at school but parents at home themselves demonstrate by their own lives that a different kind of family, whether single-parent or two-parent, is not just a possibility, but an existing reality for a particular child. How will such a child ever survive? What will become of 'family values'? It is true, as the opponents have to concede, that in the UK the Children Act of 1975 specifically provided for the adoption of children by single people, male or female; and by 'single' was here intended 'not married', so lesbian women or homosexual men would fall into this category, whether they did or did not cohabit with their partners. The children deemed suitable for such adoption, however, were those who had shown themselves to be unable to flourish in an ordinary family, who might have great difficulty in relating to more than one person at a time, and who in general were in a fairly fragile or precarious mental state by the time they came up for adoption. So this concession on the part of the adoption law would not do much to reassure those who would argue that necessarily the interests of a child of homosexual parents must be harmed.

As I have said, it is easy to be lulled into complacency by the rhetoric of 'the good of the child'. It sounds like a firm basis for moral judgement. But moral judgements, though they may and indeed should be passionately felt, ought none the less to be based on evidence or experience. And evidence about what happens to the children of homosexual parents is, understandably, almost entirely lacking. Nor is it very easy to think of illuminating analogies. If, following some members of the Christian Churches, you believe homosexuality to be a sin (and this was plainly Lady Young's view, when she led the debate on Clause 28), then it would follow that a child brought up to see nothing wrong with it might be like a child brought up in a household of thieves, who would take thieving for granted, and probably become a thief himself at an early age. Certainly people may indulge in homosexuality, or have strong homosexual leanings, because of the environment in which they find themselves for the time being, on board a ship on a long spell at sea, for example, or during endless terms at a single-sex boarding school. But this need not entail either a life-long commitment or a settled leaning towards homosexuality. It is generally believed, by people who hold to no religious dogma on the matter, that sexual orientation is not usually a matter of choice (as any sin must necessarily be, if it is to be morally condemned), but of an inborn tendency, which may take some time to manifest itself, or may be long suppressed. If this view of the matter is right, then, while a child might literally inherit some 'homosexual genes' from the one of her parents to whom she is genetically related, and therefore might possibly find herself with some homosexual tendency, she is unlikely to be so much influenced by her environment alone that she finds herself a homosexual in opposition to her natural instincts.

It could, after all, be argued that there is something potentially damaging in the situation of any child who has been born by means of AID or surrogacy, whether or not her parents are homosexual. There is an asymmetry built into the family relationships: only one of her two parents is biologically related to her, the other, though legally a parent, is not 'really' so. In this respect, it is argued, adoption is preferable to this kind of 'artificial' family. For in adopting a child, both parents are in the same boat; both have committed themselves to bringing up a child who is biologically not their own. There is no temptation for the non-related parent to blame all the child's unattractive characteristics on the other parent, whose biological offspring she partly is. In a family that has been created by assisted reproduction, there may be a danger that the parent who is not related to the child except legally may feel jealous of the other parent or inadequate in relation to the child; this does not occur in families with adopted children. However, there is no reason to suppose that such asymmetry would be more damaging in the case of homosexual than heterosexual 'parents'.

Openness

These days, no one is likely to conceal from a child that he or she is adopted, if only because children have the legal right to try to find their biological parents when they reach the age of eighteen. In the case of children born by AID, however, where the donor of semen must, according to the present UK law, have his anonymity protected, there may be a temptation to conceal the facts, though certain non-identifying information about the donor is available to the parents. Indeed, in a study of children born with the help of donors that covered the UK, Italy, the Netherlands, and Spain, published as *The European Study of Assisted Reproduction Families*, it emerged that although just over half the mothers had told a friend or family member about the method of conception of her child, not one had told the child himself. Only 12 per cent of the mothers planned to tell the child in the future, and 75 per cent had decided never to do so. Similarly, though the legal parents of a child born through surrogacy will know the identity of the birthmother, the child may never be told even that there was such a person. Such concealment of the facts of a child's birth seems intrinsically wrong, though, astonishingly, as recently as the 1970s the British Medical Association's advice to women seeking AID was to go home after treatment and forget it, or even to have sexual intercourse with the infertile husband immediately, so that if a pregnancy is achieved, it will not be absolutely clear that the husband is not, after all, the father of the child. Their pamphlet ends with the words 'No one need ever know'. This seems to me a blatant case of neglecting the 'good of the child'. The child was to be brought up in a cloud of deception: she was to know neither the identity of her father, nor that her father was a donor.

The main argument against identifying the donor is the fear that in future donors will not come forward, anxious that they will have to take some responsibility for those children whom they have fathered by AID. But in those Scandinavian countries where donor anonymity is no longer preserved, after an initial drop, the number of donors has now stabilized. Though at the time of the report of the Committee of Inquiry I was persuaded by the argument that the supply of donors would dry up if anonymity were not preserved, I now think differently. I am convinced that the law should be changed, so that children born with the help of donors would be entitled to have identifying information about the donor, as adopted children have with regard to their biological parents.

It seems only right that a child should be able to learn facts about what kind of a person the donor was. The more we know about genes, the more we may crave to know about our genetic parents. Moreover such a change would have the great advantage that they could not be kept in the dark about their conception by donor. 'By Donor' should appear on their birth certificate. It is undermining to any relationship between two people if one knows a salient fact about the other which is not divulged. Children are extremely quick to pick up signs that there is some mystery about their birth. People who know no better are likely to exclaim about characteristics of the child for which they can see no genetic explanation. Apparently innocent exclamations—'I can't think where he got all that curly hair from'—may cause such embarrassment to the parents that the child begins to smell a rat. If he accidentally discovers the truth, he may feel diminished. He will be anxious about his own identity once he discovers that, in an important sense, he is not who he thought he was. Moreover, he was not trusted with the information he may feel he was all along entitled to: he has been used by his parents to conceal their infertility, or simply as an instrument by which to satisfy their craving to be like other people and have a child.

I believe that all such deception is an evil. It is also a burden to the supposed father, who has to keep up the deception. I have been told by such a father that when he and his wife at last told their son the facts he felt a great weight lifted from his shoulders, and so did the boy, who said, 'I knew there was something funny, but I thought it was my mother'. And because it arises largely out of conventional and timid attitudes, it is, I would suggest, far less likely to be indulged in the case of homosexual parents who use AID or surrogacy to have their children. After all, in order to go down that road, they must already have decided to abandon convention, declare their determination to have a child otherwise than through the institution of heterosexual marriage or partnership, and present to the world a picture of a new sort of family, based no doubt on love, but on the love that dares, indeed demands, to speak its name.

This may constitute another possible harm to the child. As long as public attitudes to homosexuality are either to condemn it as sin, or, in the case of many school-children, to ridicule and despise it, then the children of known homosexual parents may be subject to bullying, both from adults and from other children. It could be argued that there are so many unorthodox forms of the family these days, with multiple marriages, and various kinds of single or semi-detached parents, that a few homosexuals thrown in will not make any difference. But I think genuine acceptance of homosexuals is still quite a long way off, and as long as the belief that they are sinners, or in some way seriously less than human, persists, even below the level of consciousness, then I think homosexuals who not only 'come out', but go even further and bring up children with a partner of the same sex, may be giving those children a hard time. But children are resilient, and adapt amazingly well to what outsiders may think of as bizarre or damaging circumstances. There is no evidence that these children will be permanently damaged.

Why do homosexuals want children?

It is almost inevitable that one should raise the question of the motive of homosexuals who seek assisted reproduction. Why do they want to have children? If, as must surely sometimes be the case, their motive is at least partly political — to make a point about 'gay rights', or as a feminist gesture, to prove that women do not need men — then the child they have is being used for their interests, or for the interests of their campaign, and this is a poor basis for family life. Yet this may not be a completely clear-cut argument. Many homosexuals, both men and women, see themselves, justly, as unusually loving and sympathetic people, the very kind of people who will understand and cherish a child. And if we raise the question of motivation in their case, perhaps we should raise it in the case of everyone who seeks assisted conception. Why do they need to have children? As we saw, it is not entirely easy to answer this question.

Some teenage single mothers undoubtedly want children, and if they accidentally or carelessly become pregnant do not contemplate abortion because they want, at some level of consciousness, to have someone to love and care for who will, at least for the time being, love them in return and be uncritically dependent on them. Some of these young single mothers may have a record of almost total inadequacy at school and have no ambition; through parenthood, it may seem to them that they have achieved something. The baby in the buggy is their creation, and now is their possession. (These young single mothers are the most likely to conceive again, and have another baby while they are still in their teens.) Such motives are entirely intelligible. But one could argue that here, too, the baby is being used for selfish ends. Yet neither these young single mothers nor the homosexuals we have been discussing may fail in love for their children, difficult though their circumstances may be. In neither case does it seem to me that they are deliberately inflicting injury on their children, though it may turn out that the children suffer. But we do not know that they will. So, just as there can be no law to prevent teenage girls from getting pregnant, so there can be no law based on the good of the child principle to prohibit homosexuals from making arrangements to have children. If they are turned away automatically from fertility clinics, they will proceed on their own, none the less. And this is a more hazardous course, and will, as I have said, make it inevitable that the practice remains shrouded in secrecy. This in turn will ensure that judgements of its morality or otherwise will continue to be based on ignorance.

The natural and the unnatural

Yet I am well aware that even among those who do not adopt the full-blown Sodom and Gomorrah attitude to homosexuality, there will be many who still feel profoundly uneasy at the thought that homosexuals might be permitted to establish families and bring them up, and might even be encouraged to do so through regular licensed clinics, rather than going ahead without medical help and the assurances that this would provide. For those who feel this unease, the most ready explanation is that such arrangements are contrary to nature. Is this objection a sound basis for moral condemnation?

We are faced here with a complex question. Is to say that something is unnatural the same as to say that it is wrong? (Of course if homosexual families are wrong, no one can claim a right to establish them.) David Hume, in the third book of the *Treatise of Human Nature*, dealt with the question pretty briskly. In his search for some general principle upon which, as he put it, 'all our notions of morals are founded', he declared, 'Should it be asked whether we ought to search for these notions in Nature, or whether we must look for them in some other origin, I would reply that our answer to this question depends upon the definition of the word Nature, than which there is none more ambiguous and equivocal.' In this he is right. After offering various examples of how 'the natural' is sometimes opposed to 'the artificial', sometimes to 'the usual' or 'normal', he agreeably adds that what is natural is sometimes opposed to what is miraculous 'in which sense every event that has ever happened in the world (excepting of course those miracles on which our religion is founded) is natural; so in saying that something is natural we make no very extra-ordinary discovery.' Adapting Hume's ironic remark to the present world of medical technology, we might agree that, unless we believe in miracles, it is impossible to conceive that the laws of nature may be defied, and thus whatever can now be done by new technologies, however complex, is in accordance with the laws of nature. This would, how-ever, be to use the word in so broad a sense that nothing would be contrary to nature. To see whether there is any meaning in the claim that what is unnatural is wrong, we must leave room for at least some things to be meaning-fully described as unnatural. We need to identify a concept of nature that has some content if we are to understand and assess those arguments against interventions that rely on this concept.

We may note that one of the things to which Hume thought that the natural might be opposed is the artificial. In 1983 Robert Snowden and Duncan Mitchell wrote a study of couples seeking AID to remedy their infertility entitled *The Artificial Family*. And this expression has been commonly used since for any family that has been established by the techniques of assisted conception.

Obviously the concept of artificiality is incorporated in the very expression AID. The word 'artificial' generally has a derogatory sense, though not necessarily powerfully so; it may suggest a second-best, or, more worryingly, an attempt to pass something off for what it is not. In my childhood, for example, there used to be a despised material out of which cheap clothes could be made called artificial silk. Snowden and Mitchell would certainly not have denied the derogatory overtones of the word, in the context of the family: they pointed to many difficulties and hazards in having children by AID, both in the relationship of the parents one to another, and in their relationship with the child. I have mentioned some of these dangers already. If the couple using AID, or AID combined with surrogacy, are homosexuals, then it might be supposed that the artificiality of the family, and with it the contrast with the natural, would be increased. But, as I have already suggested, this may not actually be the case. For the element of 'passing off', pretending that this was a 'natural' family, would actually be less likely than with a heterosexual family. Couples, male or female, who are overtly homosexual and are bringing up a child, cannot pretend that they acquired the child by the normal means. Nor, as I have already remarked, is it likely that they would want to.

Perhaps the contrast we are looking for, then, is between the natural and the unusual. Of this distinction Hume says 'in this sense of the word, which is the common one, there may often arise disputes concerning what is natural or unnatural; and one may in general affirm that we are not possess'd of any very precise standards by which these disputes can be decided.' For what is usual or normal, he explains, is relative to how many examples we have observed. However, we may think that Hume is here being a bit disingenuous. For the words 'normal' and 'abnormal' are not, like 'usual' and 'unusual', wholly statistical, as he would have us believe, any more than are the words 'natural' and 'unnatural' themselves. When homosexuality used to be referred to as 'unnatural vice', this did not convey merely that it was not usual, or did not conform to the norm. 'Unnatural' belongs with 'abnormal' as meaning something more than 'unusual'; more, it may be said, and worse.

So what is it about the natural that draws us to it so strongly, and especially what is it about the unnatural that repels? As we have seen from Hume, the moralist's appeal to what is natural and unnatural has always been a powerful rhetorical device; but it is especially prevalent today in arguments about the morality or otherwise of the applications of biotechnology. In 2000, Prince Charles delivered a Reith Lecture in which he rebuked biologists for drawing society into areas which 'belonged to God and God alone'. He urged them to restrict themselves to coming to understand nature, if they so wished, without trying to change it. This lecture drew an enthusiastic response from many people. He was speaking especially about genetic manipulation of crops and animals, but what he said might be generalized to cover any dramatic intervention into natural processes, including the fertilization of egg and sperm outside the human body, in the laboratory, and artificial insemination for homosexual women. Prince Charles is no fool. He did not need his father or his sister to point out, as they did, that human beings had been interfering with nature as long as they had sown crops for their own use or bred cattle for milk or meat. It cannot therefore be intervention itself that is held to be unnatural in the derogatory sense. Prince Charles allowed, as of course he had to, that agriculture and animal husbandry are not, in one sense, 'natural'. Indeed AID for breeding desired forms of cattle has been practised since the beginning of the seventeenth century. But he contrasted bad with good intervention, the latter using methods that have stood the test of time because 'they are working with the grain of nature'.

It might well be argued that new methods of remedying infertility, even IVF, though it could not have been imagined a century ago, are in one sense not in the least natural, because of the considerable intervention involved, but have been, by now, tried and tested, and are 'working with the grain of nature'. After all, it is natural that heterosexual couples should want to reproduce; and IVF may be used to help them fulfil this natural desire, if they happen to be infertile. For such couples to have children is, presumably, the way nature's grain goes. So what about AID in cases of infertility in which the husband has a very low sperm count or is incapable of intercourse? Since, as I have said, AID has been used in cattle for many years, and has been accepted as a useful procedure in an agricultural context, it surely cannot be against the grain of nature to use it to overcome human male infertility in this way? If we come to the question at issue, however—whether it is acceptable for intervention to be used to bring it about that homosexuals have children—this might be judged unhesitatingly to be against the grain of nature. It is not what normally happens.

It is clear from the above examples that accepting what goes with the grain and rejecting what goes against the grain of nature does not provide an independent criterion of acceptability. It does no more than repeat in different words the argument that would rule out intervening to allow homosexuals to have children on the grounds that it is unnatural that they should.

The search for security

I believe that the objection to some procedures on the grounds that they are unnatural is the expression of a deep-rooted fear, or rather two interconnected fears. The first arises out of the expansion and development of the biological sciences. From the mid-eighteenth century, nature began to be studied and categorized systematically. The Swedish biologist Linne (or Linnaeus), who died in 1778, with his colleagues and pupils undertook the complete classification of natural kinds, plants, birds, and animals, and these classifications, with their Latinate names, became generally accepted all over Europe. Although in a sense these classifications were recognized as artificial, they were not arbitrary, and the artifice was rather like that of grammar, rendering coherent and intelligible distinctions that were already in existence, and providing rules or laws as a framework for understanding. This meant that increasingly nature came to be regarded as a proper subject of study for the scientifically inclined, with man as observer, not needing to think in terms of the uses to which he could put his observations. The objective science of biology was beginning to emerge.

Then, not out of a clear blue sky, but against this increasingly scientific backdrop, came Darwin and his *The Origin of Species*, published in 1859. Ever since the days of Newton, philosophers, most notably Kant, had been obliged to face the problem of how human freedom, and thus of course human morality, could be reconciled with the fact that everything in the universe could be reduced to its physical components, and was governed by laws that in principle made every change predictable. What was new in the second half of the nineteenth century was the idea of historical laws of development as ineluctable as the laws of physics. *The Origin of Species* provided a theoretical explanation of how, historically, evolution occurred, through the competition for life in a world of scarcity, and the survival of the fittest. Darwin did not discuss the origin of man in this book; but when, in 1871, he published *The Descent of Man*, the biological foundation was laid for a concept of human nature which to a large extent is still with us.

However, Darwin's theory was still less than wholly explanatory. For it was not clear how the variations within a species which led some to survive and develop and others to fail actually came about. The theory at the time was that heredity worked through a kind of blending of characteristics from each parent to create something that was intermediate in the offspring. But if this were the case, it was difficult to see how parental characteristics did not simply get confused or watered down in the offspring. It was not until the 1860s, when Gregor Mendel, working on his peas in the garden of the monastery in Brünn, discovered that characteristics such as the size of a plant or the colour of its flower were passed on as separate units competing with each other for dominance, that an understanding of the mechanism of inheritance became possible. In fact, Mendel's work was overlooked until the beginning of the twentieth century, when the science of genetics, with its own laws, was formed.

It was inevitable that Darwinism and its later development into the science of genetics should face fierce opposition from theologians. Natural Theology held that the complexities and beauties of the natural world could not have come about otherwise than by the design of a Creator: it is to this tradition that Prince Charles appealed when he spoke in his lecture of interference with things that belong to God and God alone.

But, paradoxically, the more secular society becomes, the more the regularities of the natural world are necessary for its security. The fear of crossing species boundaries, for example of developing animal organs for use in human organ transplant, is a deep-rooted fear of going 'against the grain of nature'. It seems to me highly likely that, when the time comes that genetically modified pigs can be bred to provide organs for human transplant that will not be rejected by the recipients' immune systems, there will be a public outcry. Although people may learn at school, or know in theory, that men and other animals, and indeed vegetables, share numbers of genes, they will take time to know it in their hearts and accept the proposition that the boundaries between one species and another are not absolute. To cross gender boundaries is equally contrary to natural law. It is a natural law that in mammals, as opposed to vegetables, reproduction occurs by intercourse between male and female, the female giving birth, and, at least for a time, having the task of protecting the offspring. Such law should not be infringed. (It would be even more horrendous if the reported experiments in France some years ago to enable a male, by surgical intervention, to acquire a false uterus and to embark on a pregnancy became a feasible option for homosexual men.)

We are frequently reminded that we live in a 'plural' society, and that ideas of right and wrong cannot be derived from universally applicable divine commands. With divine law removed, the laws of nature seem more than ever necessary, a prop to cling to. Those whose faith rests on science rather than on God may be as alarmed as the religious to see their security removed. That homosexuals should be encouraged to reproduce may seem like the crossing of a boundary that ought to remain unbreachable.

This, then, is one source of fear. The second, connected fear has its origins in the Romantic Movement, which was more or less contemporary with the rise of the biological sciences in the late eighteenth and the nineteenth century. Rousseau's novel *Emile*, published in 1762, begins with the words 'Everything is good as it comes from the hands of the Author of Nature, but everything degenerates in the hands of man.' Here is, perhaps, another source of Prince Charles's idea that there are things best left alone by man, things which belong to God alone. Rousseau was talking about education, about how the child, in his natural state at birth, is subsequently corrupted by the intervention of conventional

teachers. But Rousseau's belief in the rightness of the natural, and the wrongness of the alienation from nature that
over-sophistication may bring, has far wider implications.

In the poets and artists of the Romantic age, we discover
the view not only that nature inspires us with our deepest
insights, but that it is itself possessed of truths to be felt and
understood only by the human imagination. And these are
truths about humanity as well as about the natural world: the
two cannot be separated. Samuel Taylor Coleridge, cha-
melion as he was, appeared capable both of adopting the
newly objective scientific stance and of expressing many of
these human-centred thoughts about nature, not only in his
poems but also in numerous entries in his notebooks.
Indeed, his notebooks and letters form a commentary on
these two parallel attitudes. On the one hand, he wrote, in a
letter to Fenwick, 'Never to see or describe any interesting
appearance in nature without connecting it by dim analogies
to the moral world proves faintness of impression. Nature has
her proper interest; and he will know what it is who believes
and feels that everything has a life of its own.' On the other
hand, there is a passage in the notebooks dated 14 April
1805 in which he expresses what seems to sum up his
thoughts, as well as those of Wordsworth and other Roman-
tics, about the peculiarly human significance of natural
objects. He writes, 'In looking at the objects of Nature while I
am thinking, as at yonder moon dim-glimmering through
the dewy window pane, I seem rather to be seeking, as it were
asking, a symbolic language for something within me that
already and forever exists than observing anything new. Even

when that latter is the case, I still always have an obscure feeling as if that new phenomenon were the dim awakening of a forgotten or hidden truth of my inner nature.' This is the true voice of Romanticism. Nature is significant. It means something other than itself. Because of man's lofty aspirations, searchings after truth, insatiable desire to understand, nature is his teacher and guide. The Romantic imagination essentially felt at one with nature, with weather, seasons, and time. Writing about his wife, Mary, in the *Prelude*, Wordsworth refers to her as 'Nature's inmate'. In the 'Lines Written a Few Miles above Tintern Abbey' there occurs an expression of something very close to what the ecologist James Lovelock has referred to as the Gaia hypothesis, that the Earth is a unified, living ecosystem, including human beings within it:

> And I have felt
> A presence that disturbs me with the joy
> Of elevated thoughts; a sense sublime
> Of something far more deeply interfused
> Whose swelling is the light of setting suns,
> And the round ocean, and the living air,
> And the blue sky, and in the mind of man,
> A motion and a spirit, that impels
> All thinking things, all objects of all thought,
> And rolls through all things.

I do not suggest that we all, or even some of us, subscribe to a belief in the Gaia hypothesis (about whose ramifications I am indeed quite ignorant). Nevertheless, when we think about nature, the word carries baggage from the Romantic age, and we cannot wholly rid ourselves of it. Nor do I believe we would want to, for many of our most profound pleasures, both in the natural world and in art, derive from this way of seeing and experiencing.

So if some course of action is, without much analysis yet readily, thought of as 'unnatural', as is medical intervention to enable homosexuals to have children, then this immediately carries with it the fear that we are alienating ourselves from what ought to be our dwelling, from the place where we want to be at home. I do not think that either of these two kinds of fear can be denied.

Is fear a proper basis for moral judgement?

But if these fears are acknowledged, do they form a proper basis for a moral judgement? Is the 'unnatural' wrong because we designate it so out of fear? I do not think so. I believe that we ought to face our fears, and recognize them for what they are: the fear of losing our certainty about natural laws by allowing everything that is possible to be tried; and the fear of losing touch with nature as it is, of alienating ourselves from that of which we as human beings form a part. We should not deny or ridicule, or otherwise attempt to dismiss, such fears. Why would we want to? But we should not deny homosexuals the children that some of them want simply on the basis that we feel nervous. Nor should we fall back on saying that they are to be denied for the sake of the children they might have. We simply do not know whether such children will be damaged. At least if we encourage homosexuals who want children to go through the procedures openly, in licensed fertility clinics, then with luck it will be possible to keep a record of their children, and in time a body of evidence will grow up on which we might be able to base a moral judgement one way or the other, and the good of the child might thereby become a concept that has some content. In any case, I doubt whether the number of homosexuals seeking to have children will be so great as to overwhelm society. There will always be more people who want to start a more usual sort of family.

Conclusions so far

So far we seem to have reached the position that while no one can properly claim a legal right to assisted conception, still less a right actually to succeed in having a child, yet the principle of compassion which generally governs the behaviour of the medical profession demands that the infertile be treated if they want to conceive. To this general rule there might be a few exceptions, but each would have to be argued and explained on its merits. These were my interim conclusions. Subsequently, I argued that there is no overriding moral objection to treating those who are not infertile, whether they seek assisted conception for reasons of convenience (the busy ballerina), or because they do not wish to tangle with the opposite sex. I suggested further that while most people may immediately regard the thought of homosexuals of either sex having children as 'unnatural', the fears underlying the use of this expression do not constitute a moral imperative to prohibit it. Society would be wrong, in my view, if it criminalized consultants or clinics that provided assisted conception to homosexuals. If resources are scarce, it is right that the infertile should have priority over the others: they, after all, plainly have 'something wrong with them'. In any case, it seems wrong that limited resources should be used for those who seek assistance just for their own convenience, or to set up their own preferred single-sex families. Nevertheless, provided they are prepared to pay, I do not believe that it should be either for doctors or for society at large to prevent individual homosexuals from bringing up their own, or partly their own, children. There is no evidence that harm will come of it, or that it will prove contrary to the common good. It is important in such matters to distinguish between offence (which may be caused to some) and harm.

Are all methods of fertility treatment legitimate?

It is time now to address the question of whether there are some methods of assisted conception that are themselves intrinsically wrong, whatever the gender or sexual orientation of those who might seek them. I listed at the beginning the most usual procedures used to provide assistance in conception, but deferred discussion of the two methods that are most morally dubious. The first of these is surrogacy. Surrogacy is the commissioning of a woman to carry a baby whom she has agreed to give up at the end of the pregnancy. It is an essential part of the enterprise of a male homosexual's having a child. It may also be a remedy for a heterosexual couple who want to have a child, where the woman, let us say, has no uterus or, after repeated miscarriages, is deemed unable to sustain a pregnancy, perhaps for no apparent reason. Or it might be that the general health of a woman, while good enough for her to be able to look after a child, would put her at risk if she became pregnant. Is surrogacy, then, an acceptable remedy for certain sorts of infertility; and, if so, is it also acceptable as part of the process of allowing homosexuals to become fathers?

This was one of the issues on which the Committee of Inquiry into Human Fertilisation and Embryology found itself unable to agree. The 1990 Act is equally half-hearted and prevaricating. There were those on the Committee who argued that since a surrogacy arrangement could be set up privately, without reference to doctors or lawyers (for the surrogate mother could be impregnated either using the would-be father's semen to inject herself, or by sexual intercourse with the would-be father), it would be better if there were a system by which such arrangements could be regulated, and where, in the case of an infertile couple at least, a consultant could advise and supervise the proceedings. In some cases where, for example, the female partner could produce eggs, but could not sustain a pregnancy, her eggs could be fertilized with her partner's sperm, and the surrogate could become pregnant through IVF. And so the child the surrogate mother handed over would not be her biological child at all. She would simply be lending her womb as a living incubator. This could not be done without medical intervention.

A minority of the Committee thought, therefore, that there should be an official non-profit-making surrogacy agency, rather like an adoption agency, through which surrogacy arrangements could be made. This agency would lay down, for example, what expenses should be paid to the surrogate, and the terms and conditions under which the child should be handed over to the parents who were to bring it up. I have come to think that probably this minority was right. However, the majority thought that to set up such an agency would be to condone surrogacy, a practice they regarded as intrinsically wrong, and likely to lead to trouble, if not to disaster, for all the parties involved, including the child. It may be that the view of the majority was over-influenced by the fact that, at the time, there were numerous stories in circulation about highly profitable commercial surrogacy agencies in the United States, and off-shoots of such agencies appeared poised to establish themselves in the UK, advertising for surrogates and sending out their particulars to would-be users, often in glaringly sexist terms, with fees to be paid through the agency. All this seemed to some on the Committee, including myself, extra-ordinarily exploitative of the women involved. Even though they might have chosen to act as surrogates, the motives of these women would have been commercial, and the whole enterprise seemed to trivialize and vulgarize childbirth.

Even before the main Human Fertilisation and Embryology legislation in 1990, a Bill was rushed through Parliament to prohibit the setting up of any such commercial agency in the UK. In the subsequent legislation, though to enter into a surrogacy arrangement did not become a criminal offence, no contract entered into by a surrogate and a commissioning couple, or single man, was to be legally enforceable. Thus, if, as might well happen, the mother who gave birth to the child changed her mind when the child was born and refused to hand it over, the commissioning couple would have no remedy in law. Refusal to part with the baby was much more likely if the child was genetically related to the birth-mother, as it would be in the case of surrogacy undertaken on behalf of a homosexual man. So the position remains ambiguous.

There is no doubt that surrogacy is an extremely risky enterprise, and liable to end in tears. In the decade or so since legislation there have been numerous surrogacies arranged (those who had argued in favour of proper regulation had urged the fact that the practice would go on anyway, and they were right); doubtless many have gone smoothly, though we have no way of telling what effect they have had on either child or surrogate mother, or indeed the commissioner of the arrangement. But the press delight in the stories of failures, of couples who refuse to accept a child who is born with some defect, or of birth-mothers who refuse to surrender the child, or of commissioning couples who simply decide they do not want a child after all or get divorced before the child is born. There are numerous ways in which such a precarious arrangement can fail. The question of anonymity, for example, is far more complex than in the case of AID, where the identity of the donor is, according to present UK law, not known even to the parents (though, as I have explained, I believe that the law ought to be changed on this point). In the case of surrogacy, the commissioning parents or parent will undoubtedly know the identity of the surrogate, and often close relations have been established during the pregnancy. Indeed, sometimes the surrogate who gives birth entertains the hope that she may be able to keep in touch with the baby, or even have a special role in its life. This is always a dangerous and vain hope, unless the surrogate is, say, a sister bearing the child for her infertile sibling out of kindness.

There are several organizations in the UK that exist to put couples, heterosexual or homosexual, in touch with surrogates, but these are not full-blown profit-making companies, and therefore do not quite fall foul of the law. But, though such organizations may raise expectations that a surrogate can be found, and though to some extent they have a duty to attempt to find one (that is their *raison d'être*), none may be forthcoming. No legal right will have been infringed, and probably no moral right either.

In fact, the present position in the UK with regard to surrogacy is thoroughly confused, and there is understandably a good deal of dissatisfaction with it. For example, a surrogate is supposed, like the donor of sperm, to be paid 'expenses only', not a fee which might induce her to do something she might turn out to wish she had not undertaken, or exploit her if she is vulnerable through poverty. But, while it may be possible to work out a reasonable scale of expenses for a young man to come to hospital for an hour or two to give sperm, the expenses that may accrue from pregnancy are not so easy to calculate. There may be loss of earnings, there will certainly be new clothes, and there will be equipment for the baby when it is born. 'Expenses' might turn into something pretty substantial. Certainly one former surrogate appeared on UK television some time ago and boasted that she had been able to recarpet her house on the proceeds, and this was why she had undertaken the arrangement. It is hard not to feel a certain revulsion for so detached and apparently inhuman an attitude to childbearing. But if there are those who can adopt it, and if there are others who genuinely want the service, then perhaps one can say no more than that it would be impossible for most people to contemplate such an arrangement, unless perhaps between close friends or sisters, where the fertile woman felt so deep a compassion for the infertile that she was prepared to bear a child and hand it over. Such sentiment does not amount to a moral argument, one way or the other. At any rate, if the earlier argument is to be accepted, that there should be no law prohibiting homosexual men from bringing up children whose genetic fathers they are, then it is necessary, if one is to be consistent, to allow that surrogacy cannot be prohibited either. But I now believe that it would be better if the process were officially regulated, and more openly discussed between doctors, prospective parents, surrogates, and, later, with the resulting children.

It is perhaps pertinent to raise a quite general question in the context of surrogacy, though it has application elsewhere among the issues that have been discussed. On the whole, the attitude of the USA seems to be that if there is a market for something like surrogacy then that shows that it is what people want, and it is perfectly reasonable to satisfy the demand. It is as good a way of making money as any other 'niche market'. The fact that a number of people do not like the idea of hiring out surrogate mothers is entirely irrelevant. No one is forced either to become a surrogate or to make use of one. When the hasty legislation to which I have already referred was rushed through in the UK at the end of a Parliamentary session in 1989, it was passed through Parliament on a wave of revulsion against anything so vulgar and exploitative as the American commercial companies who were hovering on the shores of Britain. The general sentiment was 'not in our back yard'. If people wanted to enter into surrogacy contracts, let them go across the Atlantic to do it. I do not remember any very serious discussion of whether or not surrogacy was intrinsically so immoral, or its consequences so socially disastrous, that legislation against it must be enacted. No one could dislike the idea of for-profit surrogacy agencies more than I do. And I am certainly aware of all the ways that surrogacy arrangements can go wrong. Yet I increasingly believe that one social ill we need to beware of is that of excessive governmental regulation. If surrogacy were allowed in the UK, on the American model, though some people might be offended, I doubt if we would be harmed; nor would it constitute a creeping and insidious damage to British society, like the increase in the carrying of firearms or the spread of juvenile alcoholism. After all, surrogate contracts are fairly specialist things. I am not sure, but I suspect, that the legislation hastened through at the time of the Committee of Inquiry into Human Fertilisation and Embryology was mistaken. It has certainly left the possible moral arguments, including arguments about whether people have a right to make surrogacy arrangements if they want to, in a state of confusion.

Finally, there is another technique that could in principle one day be used to remedy certain kinds of infertility, when a man has become sterile through cancer treatment, say, or a woman has no uterus or cannot produce eggs. This is cloning. Cloning is a form of nonsexual reproduction in which all the offspring are genetically identical to each other and to the parent from which they are derived. All the identical organisms, parent and offspring, are collectively a clone; and each individual in the group is a clone of all the others. Many plants, such as strawberries, reproduce both sexually by seeds and also by putting out suckers that produce plants that are simply extensions of the parent plant. Human beings have long interfered with nature by forming clones of plants by cuttings. Thus all the Bramley Seedling apples in the world are clones of one original parent.

Mammals can clone naturally, by a quite different process, when a single embryo divides in the uterus to form identical twins (or, with two divisions, identical quadruplets). But it takes radical intervention to produce the clone of a mammal in any other way.

Research has been going on for many years to investigate the possibility of artificially cloning animals, with a view to providing a quick way to reproduce a particularly successful strain of cattle or sheep. Fifty years ago the biologist John Gurden, working both in Oxford and Cambridge, took the nuclei out of frogs' eggs and transferred intestinal cells from an adult frog into the egg to replace its own nucleus, and succeeded in developing tadpoles. These tadpoles did not, however, develop into frogs. But later, using cells from tadpoles to transfer to the eggs, he succeeded in cloning tadpoles that did grow to maturity. However, it is much easier to work with frogs and salamanders, which have large eggs and where fertilization and development takes place outside the body, than with mammals; for some time it was believed that mammalian cloning was impossible. And then, in 1997, an announcement was made of the birth of Dolly, a sheep that had been successfully cloned by scientists at the Roslin Institute outside Edinburgh. This was a genuine breakthrough.

The method used to produce Dolly was to take a mammary cell from an adult ewe (a Finn Dorset variety) and culture it in the laboratory, so that it multiplied. Meanwhile, an egg was harvested from another ewe (a Scottish Blackface) and its nucleus was extracted using a pipette. The whole cell from the first ewe was then inserted into the 'shell' of the egg, and, by means of a brief exposure to an electric current, the egg fused to form a reconstructed embryo. However, the resulting embryo did not have DNA completely identical to that of the Finn Dorset ewe from which the cells had been taken because it still had a small amount of the DNA belonging to the Scottish Blackface, that contained in the mitochondrial cells which continued to line the 'shell' of her egg. So, in fact, a clone formed by nuclear transfer, unlike clones formed naturally from the division of the embryo, though its genes come predominantly from the animal from whom the cells were originally taken, also inherits a small but significant number from the female whose egg has been enucleated, and these genes pass only through the female line.

The reconstituted embryos are extremely fragile, and transferring them to the uterus of the surrogate mother who is to carry them to term is a matter of great difficulty. At Roslin the scientists produced 277 reconstructed embryos, and transferred twenty-nine of them, those that seemed to be in good condition, into thirteen surrogate mothers, and produced only one viable lamb as a result. However, much has happened since then, and techniques will doubtless be improved with experience.

As soon as Dolly's birth was announced, the inevitable question arose: if sheep, why not humans? To which the immediate answer was that the risks were far too great. It is inconceivable that any experimentation could be carried out that involved so many surrogates, and so many failures, if the subjects were people. And experimentation is what it would be; for no one could consider it as treatment with so extremely uncertain an outcome. Moreover, it is not yet established what effect being a clone may have on an animal. Dolly, unlike many of the failed sheep clones, was not deformed at birth, though rather unnaturally large. Then, however, she began to show signs of premature ageing and suffered from arthritis in her legs. She died in 2003, aged only six. I believe that the risks of human cloning would be too great for it ever to be tried in the foreseeable future. One of the worst risks would be that even if a successful baby were born, its future health would be a matter of 'waiting to see'. No mother or child could be asked to put up with this.

But let us imagine that in the future the risks become fewer, and the techniques more sure. Is there then any reason, in principle, why human cloning should not be carried out? This is a question that demands a serious answer, and I shall attempt to answer it in due course.

Cloning: 1997–2001

However, first it is necessary to say a little about what has happened to cloning since the birth of Dolly. A crucial distinction has been drawn between reproductive and therapeutic cloning. Reproductive cloning results, as in the case of Dolly, after cell nuclear transfer in the birth by a surrogate of a clone animal. Already, since the birth of Dolly, clone piglets have been born, the cells of which have been genetically modified at the nuclear transfer stage, with a view to a new possibility of using pig organs for human transplants without the risk of rejection of the transplanted organs. This is an enormous new field of research. But, with or without genetic modification, there is the possibility that the cloning of farm animals might provide a swift way of improving stock, and transforming the profitability of animal husbandry, if it could be developed into a safe and routine procedure, though there would be a risk of diminishing the gene pool for any species, a risk that could have serious consequences for the future viability and health of that species.

In humans, reproductive cloning would have as its aim the nonsexual production of a complete human baby, born to a surrogate, whether the motive for doing this was to allow a couple to have a baby at least one-sidedly genetically related to themselves (in a case where there was total male infertility, or for some other cause); or, more alarmingly, where some-one wanted to reproduce him or herself genetically, or, going further into the realms of political fantasy, where a dictator wanted to ensure that he had an army of cloned obedient guards, or persons of such low IQ and modest ambition that they would be for ever happy to sweep the roads or clean the public lavatories. Another equally socially or politically inspired aim would be to eliminate defects, whether physical or mental, from a population so as to pro-duce a 'perfect' race. This would be eugenics, on a grand scale.

Therapeutic cloning, on the other hand, uses only the first part of the technique of reproductive cloning. Embryos are created in the laboratory by the denucleating of a donated egg and the transfer of the nucleus of another cell into the shell of that egg, as with reproductive cloning. But then the cells of that newly created embryo, before they have differen-tiated into specific types of cell, are used to generate cell-lines, potentially of any type of cell that occurs in the body. It would defeat the purpose of this kind of procedure if the embryo so produced were to be allowed to develop to the stage when its cells had already differentiated into specific types of cell (that is, four or five days after the embryo was reconstituted). The whole point of the research depends on the cells of the newly created embryo being allowed to develop while they are still undifferentiated. So the interests of those engaged in research into therapeutic cloning are totally different from those of anyone, if there were anyone, interested in human reproductive cloning.

The aim of therapeutic cloning, as its name implies, is to develop cell-lines, which can be induced in the laboratory to develop from their pluripotent state into a specific type of cell, and which can go on multiplying for ever, to establish a bank of cells which, one day, may be transplanted into damaged human organs, including the brain, to repair the damage and restore function. In describing this process, I have very much simplified it, and have left out any account of the difficulties that still stand in the way of any such possibilities. Nevertheless, it is true to say that cell transplantation is not fantasy, but is something that might be developed over the next decade. Though adult stem cells may be used to develop some cell lines, they are much more limited in scope than embryonic stem cells. Most scientists believe that embryonic stem cells, taken from embryos cloned in the laboratory, are crucial to research into such new therapy, which could provide a means of restoring a brain damaged by Alzheimer's or Parkinson's disease, or a way of healing a spine damaged by injury. Regulations have now been introduced in the UK through Parliament that have extended the permissible uses of pre-fourteen-day-old embryos in research, not only in projects connected with fertility and infertility, as the original legislation stated, but also to work towards such pioneering therapy as cell transplantation, and to increase our knowledge of how the cells of the early embryo develop so that such therapy may become a reality. Following the introduction of the regulations a Select Committee was set up to examine further all the issues involved. That committee's report concluded that embryonic stem-cell research should be permitted, as far as possible using 'spare' embryos, which had come into existence as a part of IVF procedures. Meanwhile, it was thought that the scope of the new legislation, which allows live embryos to be used for research into therapeutic cloning, did not allow human reproductive cloning.

However, in November 2001, a test case was brought to the High Court by one of the pro-life groups, who were convinced that once the production of embryos by cell nuclear replacement had been allowed, human reproductive cloning would follow. They claimed that the present UK legislation did not rule out human reproductive cloning.

It had been assumed that the 1990 Act, which had specifically criminalized the creation of human clones using cells from embryos fertilized in vitro, would have covered all human cloning. But on 15 November, Mr Justice Crane ruled that embryos created by cell nuclear replacement were not covered by the Act, which refers in the relevant part to 'live human embryos where fertilization is complete'. Now in 1984, when the report of the Committee of Inquiry into Human Fertilisation and Embryology was written, and from which much of the wording of the 1990 Act was derived, the possibility of creating embryos by cell nuclear replacement (that is without the fertilization of a human egg by human sperm) was not known. It was assumed that the only way to produce an embryo was by fertilization. So, in the light of our then knowledge, the words 'where fertilization is complete' were otiose. We could have simply written 'live human embryos'. If we had done so, the Act would have covered all embryos, however produced. But with the new method of creating embryos, those produced otherwise than by fertilization were, by implication, excluded.

As soon as Mr Justice Crane gave his judgement, the excitable Professor Antinori, already mentioned in connection with his enthusiasm for making babies for postmenopausal women, announced his intention of coming to England to make use of the loophole, to be helped, as he claimed, by an English doctor and 200 women who had volunteered to act as surrogates. He boasted that there would be a cloned human baby within a year. The British Government appeared to be completely thrown by this threat, and rushed through legislation in almost less than the minimum possible time, to prohibit the insertion into a woman's uterus of an embryo created by cell nuclear replacement. The Bill went through all its stages and is now law. The more level-headed parliamentarians believed this Bill to be unnecessary: the Human Fertilisation and Embryology Authority had already said that it would not give a license to anyone proposing to attempt human reproductive cloning, which is in any case illegal elsewhere in Europe. The only advantage of the legislation as passed is that when the question of therapeutic cloning comes up for Parliamentary debate again, as it surely will, no one will be able to confuse the arguments by deploying the slippery slope as a reason against it. The slope down towards human reproductive cloning has already been blocked by primary legislation. Nobody need fear it any more.

Would the cloning of humans be intrinsically wrong?

It is time now to address the question of the morality, as opposed to the legality, of human cloning. As I have said, for the foreseeable, indeed the imaginable, future, the attempt to clone humans would be wrong on grounds of risk and uncertainty. No one should be permitted to subject their fellow humans to such risks, even if those people agree to become part of the trial. After all, those who really want children are genuinely desperate, and may be prepared to accept risks which in a more rational, less vulnerable frame of mind they would see as unacceptable. Such people should not be exploited by scientists or doctors anxious to be first in the field, and make a name for themselves (as well as probable wealth). It seems to me very likely that human cloning will never be tried, given the moral unacceptability of testing such radical procedures on human subjects. And I would be happy to accept this embargo.

But if we can contemplate the hypothetical situation in which the risks have been minimized, or even eliminated, then the question remains whether the cloning of humans should be prohibited on grounds of moral unacceptability and the moral outrage that it would provoke. Since natural clones, in the form of identical twins, exist and are not regarded with horror, it cannot be the mere fact of human beings who share identical DNA that causes the moral outrage, especially as clones produced by cell nuclear transfer would not be as completely genetically identical as naturally formed identical twins. As I have mentioned, the new cloned baby would inherit some genes from the outer shell of the egg that had been denucleated before receiving its new nucleus, the mitochondrial cells. (These, though few in number, are important, and may be the cause of serious disease if they are malformed.) So what is it about the thought of deliberately produced human clones that produces such moral horror?

Some have argued that to be born a clone would be to be born without a basic human right, namely the right to have one's own personal identity. But this is nonsense. No one believes that identical twins, being spatially and physiologically separate from each other, do not each possess personal identity. Even Siamese twins are commonly held to have distinct identities.

Some people argue that cloning would be morally wrong because only immoral people would want to have clones of themselves created. I do not believe that this is true. Some infertile men (and their wives) might deeply want a clone of themselves. The only person I have actually come across who wants to be cloned is an Australian who wrote to me (and the Prime Minister, and doubtless many others) to say that he has two surrogate mothers lined up to receive reconstructed embryos using his cells, and that he simply wants permission to go ahead. He claims that all he desires is to have sons, having become sterile in consequence of treatment for prostate cancer. He thinks he is being unreasonably denied something that is his right. Unfortunately, he is over-optimistic about the feasibility at the moment of human cloning using adult cells. And since he is already eighty-four years of age he is unlikely to live long enough to fulfil his ambition. Nevertheless, his motivation does not seem particularly sinister, nor his goals immoral. He is just a bit unrealistic.

Some assert that it would be an intolerable burden for a child, a son, say, to be the clone of his father, for he would be able to foresee exactly what he would become as he grew to his father's age. This argument seems to me to have no more force than the previous argument. The son would be brought up in a very different environment from the father, being of a different generation, and therefore with different cultural assumptions and different opportunities for development. There are already numerous sons who inherit genes from their father which they may see expressed in themselves, sometimes with dismay, such as a tendency to early baldness or an addictive personality. This does not constitute an intolerable burden, or at least it need not. We are not, any of us, nothing except our genes.

Some objectors argue that it must necessarily be wrong to allow a child to be born who is not the offspring of the fertilization of egg and sperm, and that to produce a clone by cell nuclear replacement would be to break the proper connection between a child and two parents of different gender. It is not clear to me that there is any evidence that this would be especially damaging to an individual child, or more damaging than being born by artificial means to a homosexual couple. But of course there is no such evidence at the present time. I believe, however, that this argument is not concerned with the possible effects on individuals of being born a clone: it is rather a general argument against allowing nonsexual reproduction. And it merges into what I believe are the real arguments against human cloning, which I have briefly mentioned already. These are social and political arguments. To produce a human clone seems to be the ultimate and most extreme example of the manipulation of human beings by other human beings. It is not that each individual cloned child would be deprived of free will; he would be as much free and as much determined as the rest of us, no more and no less. The fear is rather that some person, or some regime, might one day exercise such power that people could be born to their command, in the numbers they dictated, and, worst of all, with the characteristics they thought desirable. This would be to eliminate the chanciness of life and the recalcitrance of human beings, the 'twisted timber of humanity' on which democracies flourish, but which is anathema to dictatorships. For the concern that above all lies behind the fear of cloning is that, in making a clone, the genes of the newly nucleated egg may be changed, according to the purposes or preferences of the scientist or his master. This is the fear of *A Brave New World*.

It is already possible to produce cloned animals with specific characteristics introduced at the stage when the new nucleus is inserted into the egg. The year after Dolly was born the biotechnology company who were research partners at the Roslin Institute produced another cloned sheep, Polly, who was not only cloned but also genetically engineered. The cells that gave rise to Polly were fitted with a human gene that causes her to secrete a human blood-clotting factor in her milk. If this transformation can be replicated, as no doubt it can, then the benefit to haemophiliacs, who lack this factor in their blood, would be enormous. And, as I have said, the same company have produced a family of five genetically engineered piglets fitted out with the ability to prevent rejection by human beings if any of their organs were transplanted into a human body. The possibility of this kind of genetic engineering seems to have come nearer with the advent of cloned animals.

In the 1990s it seemed that it might be possible to alter the genes of a human embryo brought into existence by in vitro fertilization, before placing it in a woman's uterus. In this way, for example, an embryo could be 'cured' of a monogenetic disease before it was even born, by having the faulty gene removed or replaced. This possibility seems now to have receded, but the spectre of 'designer babies' has come back in the context of human cloning. If genetic engineering were confined to the elimination of mono-genetic diseases there would be almost no one, I suspect, who could seriously argue against it. If it could be carried out with a reasonable chance of success it would come to be regarded as a therapeutic tool which should be used to prevent suffering, both in the individual child and in the family. Those, however, who talk of 'designer babies' are thinking of babies, whether cloned or born by in vitro fertilization, who are engineered not to avoid a severe disease or disability but in order positively to come up to some sort of ideal held by their parents. I do not know how realistic this fear is, or whether it will come to seem simply a fantasy. I am certain of one thing: to allow parents to insist that their babies must be of a certain kind would be a disaster. Of anyone who wanted only a baby of the right specification one would be bound to ask about her motivation. What did she want this baby *for*? If it was to satisfy her vanity or her ambition, then the baby is truly being thought of, as is often said, as a commodity, even a fashion accessory. It is easy for young parents to think of their children as their possessions. It takes time and experience to learn that one does not own one's children, and has a very limited power over them. I have spoken of the chanciness of ordinary conception, the mixture of genes for each child being unpredictable; I have spoken of the recalcitrance of people, who will not necessarily conform to what other people want for them. Any attempt to remove these features from the enterprise of having children seems not only doomed to failure, but to be the likely cause of misery and disappointment, on the part of both the parents and the child. One can, within reason, choose the person with whom one will have a child, with whose genes one's own will be mixed, but there can be no right to choose, more specifically, what genes a child shall have (even if such a thing were to become possible). This brings us back to the fundamental objection to human cloning, whether or not the cloned child is also genetically engineered. It suggests a false idea of the control that one person may have over another.

It therefore seems that human cloning should never be allowed, except perhaps in cases of complete male infertility, when all other remedies have failed. I believe that, with this possible exception in mind, it is perhaps a pity that the UK has joined the rest of Europe in an absolute ban on such cloning. But at present there is no doubt that for various reasons, some of them confused, most people find the idea of it morally abhorrent. They will therefore have welcomed the decision of Parliament, even though given the efficient methods of licensing and control that we have in the UK, the resulting legislation may not have been strictly necessary.

A rights-based morality

I started by asking whether people had a right to have children. I distinguished, somewhat simplistically, between rights conferred by law, and rights that someone may claim though there is no law which confers them, but which they believe some vaguer concept of a moral or human law should confer. The existence of the Human Rights Act renders this distinction somewhat unclear. At any rate, it seems that the right to have a child cannot be a right in either the legal or the moral sense; for it may be impossible for some people to conceive. However, it might well be thought that a moral right exists that one should not be prevented from having a child. Is there also a right for those who are infertile that they should be given assistance to conceive by the medical profession? I, myself, would prefer to express the relation between the infertile couple and their doctor in terms of the doctor's professional duty, which is a duty of compassion to his patients, which makes it obligatory for him to seek as far as he can to alleviate suffering. The duty in question is not so much legal as moral and professional, and it arises as part of the whole deeply value-laden institution of medicine. A doctor who felt himself under no such obligation to his patients should not have entered the medical profession in the first place, and having done so is simply a bad doctor.

Does the fact that such duties as these exist entail that those who seek the help of a doctor have a right to that help? As I have already said, I do not believe that it does. Someone who is a good and conscientious teacher in a school may feel herself under a professional obligation to try to get to know her students, and as far as possible help their development and further their interests in various ways, apart from her classroom teaching, though through this as well. Her students may come to expect this from her, but to say that is different from saying that they have a right, or a definite claim on her time and energy. Looking back on her when they have left school, they may say that they feel grateful to her; and this is strongly to suggest that she did more than what they could have claimed as a right. Gratitude is out of place if you are given only what is your due. Yet she herself would say that she was doing what it was the duty of a teacher to do.

So in this sense there may be duties that are not created simply by the fact that someone has a right. Yet it is certain that there is an increasing tendency for people to base their moral judgements on some concept of rights. If this is so, it leads to a change in the relationship between doctors and their patients. As I have said, there is, or was, a deeply embedded compassion in the self-image of the doctor (even lurking in the heart of the most arrogant surgeon). And this is why rogue doctors who murder or rape their patients are so peculiarly horrifying. This compassion is intrinsically paternalistic; the doctor is in a position of superior knowledge and skill. He or she can help someone in trouble. He or she is a Good Samaritan. Many people when they or their children are ill feel themselves both ignorant and vulnerable; they seek the help of a doctor as suppliants (even if they pay him a fee). They may actually feel that they need a father or mother figure: they need to be told what is the best thing to do. This is to say that, in the best cases, there is a relationship of trust between patient and doctor.

Now, if it becomes commonly the case that patients seek treatment, even a particular kind of treatment, as a right (that they demand, say, in vitro fertilization or the provision of a surrogate) then this relationship is changed. The patient becomes a client, the doctor obliged to provide what the patient wants. The doctor becomes more like, say, a hairdresser. People may well listen to the advice of their hairdressers, and will certainly rely on the hairdresser's skill, which they do not themselves possess. But in the last resort the hairdresser is the servant of his client.

There are many who welcome this change in the status of the doctor. There is a strong move to bring patients more centrally into medical decision-making. Critics of the old relationship believe that the days of paternalism, when the doctor was a god-like figure, above questioning or criticism, are long past. And it is true that a refusal to believe that the patient had the right to any opinions, or the right to know what was going on, or to understand it, were indeed, in some cases, horrendous. The father-figure could be a bully and a dictator. Nevertheless, I should deeply regret a new system of rights within which a doctor had none but a contractual duty to carry out whatever procedures his client might demand. I should be sorry if the ethics of compassion were removed from the transaction between doctor and patient.

In any case, I believe that it is essential to the integrity of the medical profession that doctors should be allowed to say that they will not carry out a procedure demanded by a patient, on conscientious grounds. (In fact I doubt if such a situation arises often, except in the case of abortion: in the more outrageous cases, like that of causing a postmenopausal woman to have a baby, it generally becomes known that someone, a Professor Antinori, is willing to do the job. There is probably no great need for shopping around.)

We must beware of the danger of confusing what is passionately and deeply wanted with what is a right. It is good if possible, and if no harm to others ensues, to try to get people what they very much want. But if they fail to get what they want they may be disappointed, but they have not, so far, been wronged. Under the Human Rights Act, if people think they have been wronged, their human rights infringed, they may go to a tribunal, where it will be for a judge to decide between what was a strong desire and what was a right. There is no harm in this power being allocated to the judiciary. Indeed, to whom else could it belong? Judges are professionally committed to listening to pleas, and to coming to an unbiased decision on the rights and wrongs of the case. When enough case-law has been built up on such decisions, judges will have a tradition to fall back on; it will no longer seem arbitrary that the decision goes one way rather than another.

My other anxiety about the new morality, as it will come to bear on the issue of demands for assisted conception, is perhaps more nebulous, and it is one that I have hinted at already. If something is regarded as a right, however strongly you feel that it is something you want or need, as well as something that you deserve, you may come to feel less strongly about the thing itself, as you feel more strongly that you must get your due. I would deplore any tendency for people to become so much obsessed with their right to have a child, and to have it in the way they want, even with the characteristics they would prefer, that they forget the old sense of astonishment and gratitude that came with the birth of a child. Gratitude to whom? Well, to God or nature, or the midwife or the doctor, or the principle of continuity and the renewal of life itself. It does not matter. But, as I have said, gratitude is something you do not feel when all you have got is what is owed.

Index